RYPINS' INTENSIVE REVIEWS

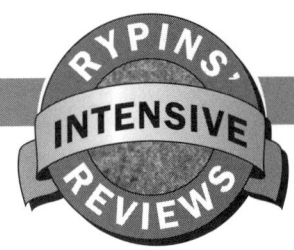

Series Editor

Edward D. Frohlich, MD

Alton Ochsner Distinguished Scientist
Vice President for Academic Affairs
Alton Ochsner Medical Foundation
Staff Member, Ochsner Clinic
Professor of Medicine and of Physiology
Louisiana State University of Medicine
Adjunct Professor of Pharmacology and
Clinical Professor of Medicine
Tulane University School of Medicine
New Orleans, Louisiana

RYPINS' INTENSIVE REVIEWS

Surgery

Ravi S. Chari, MD

Chief Resident in Surgery
Duke University Medical Center
Durham, North Carolina

David C. Sabiston, Jr., MD

James B. Duke Professor and Chairman
Department of Surgery
Duke University Medical Center
Durham, North Carolina

Lippincott - Raven
PUBLISHERS
Philadelphia • New York

Acquisitions Editor: Richard Winters
Sponsoring Editor: MaryBeth Murphy
Production Editor: Molly E. Dickmeyer
Design Coordinator: Melissa Olson
Managing Editor: Susan E. Kelly
Interior Designer: Susan Blaker
Cover Designer: William T. Donnelly
Production Service: P.M. Gordon Associates
Printer: Courier/Kendallville
Cover Printer: Lehigh Press

ISBN: 0-397-51551-0

Library of Congress Cataloging-in-Publication Data

Chari, Ravi S.
    Surgery / Ravi S. Chari, David C. Sabiston, Jr.
        p.   cm. – (Rypins' intensive reviews)
    Includes index.
    ISBN 0-397-51551-0
    1. Surgery—Outlines, syllabi, etc.   2. Surgery—Examinations,
questions, etc.   I. Sabiston, David C., 1924–   . II. Title.
III. Series.
    [DNLM: 1. Surgery—examination questions.   WO 18.2 C473s 1996]
RD37.3C48   1996
617′.0076–dc20
DNLM/DLC
for Library of Congress   96-18898
                                                                CIP

9 8 7 6 5 4 3 2 1

Preface

In this text, those aspects common to all branches of surgery (principles of surgery) are considered first. This is followed by a discussion of specific surgical lesions encountered in various organs and anatomic sites.

Ravi S. Chari, MD

Who Was "Rypins"?

Dr. Harold Rypins (1892–1939) was the founding editor of what is now known as the RYPINS' series of review books. Originally published under the title *Medical State Board Examinations,* the first edition was published by J. B. Lippincott Company in 1933. Dr. Rypins edited subsequent editions of the book in 1935, 1937, and 1939 before his death that year. The series that he began has since become the longest-running and most successful publication of its kind, having served as an invaluable tool in the training of generations of medical students. Dr. Rypins was a member of the faculty of Albany Medical College in Albany, New York, and also served as Secretary of the New York State Board of Medical Examiners. His legacy to medical education flourishes today in the highly successful *Rypins' Basic Sciences Review* and *Rypins' Clinical Sciences Review,* now in their 16th editions, and in the *Rypins' Intensive Reviews* series of subject review volumes. We at Lippincott–Raven Publishers take pride in this continuing success.

–The Publisher

▼
Series Preface

These are indeed very exciting times in medicine. Having made this statement, one's thoughts immediately reflect about the major changes that are occurring in our overall healthcare delivery system, utilization-review and shortened hospitalizations, issues concerning quality assurance, ambulatory surgical procedures and medical clearances, and the impact of managed care on the practice of internal medicine and primary care. Each of these issues has had a considerable impact on the approach to the patient and on the practice of medicine.

But even more mind-boggling than the foregoing changes are the dramatic changes imposed on the practice of medicine by fundamental conceptual scientific innovations engendered by advances in basic science that no doubt will affect medical practice of the immediate future. Indeed, much of what we thought of as having a potential impact on the practice of medicine of the future has already been perceived. One need only take a cursory look at our weekly medical journals to realize that we are practicing "tomorrow's medicine today." And consider that the goal a few years ago of actually describing the human genome is now near reality.

Reflect, then, for a moment on our current thinking about genetics, molecular biology, cellular immunology, and other areas that have impacted upon our current understanding of the underlying mechanisms of the pathophysiological concepts of disease. Moreover, paralleling these innovations have been remarkable advances in the so-called "high tech" and "gee-whiz" aspects of how we diagnose disease and treat patients. We can now think with much greater perspective about the dimensions of more specific biologic diagnoses concerned with molecular perturbations; gene therapy not only affecting genetic but oncological diseases; more specific pharmacotherapy involving highly specific receptor inhibition, alterations of intracellular signal transduction, manipulations of cellular protein synthesis; immunosuppresive therapy not only with respect to organ transplantations but also of autoimmune and other immune-related diseases; and therapeutic means for manipulating organ remodeling or the intravascular placement of stents. Each of these concepts has become inculcated into our everyday medical practice within the past decade. The reason why these changes have so rapidly promoted an upheaval in medical practice is continuing medical education, a constant awareness of the current medical literature, and a thirst for new knowledge.

To assist the student and practitioner in the review process, the publisher and I have initiated a new approach in the publication of *Rypins' Basic Sciences Review* and *Rypins' Clinical Sciences Review*. Thus, when I assumed responsibility to edit this long-standing board review series with the 13th edition of the textbook (first published in 1931), it was with a feeling of great excitement. I perceived that great changes would be coming to medicine, and I believed that this would be one ideal means of not only facing these changes head on but also for me personally to cope and keep up with these changes. Over the subsequent editions, this confidence was reassured and rewarded. The presentation for the updating of medical information was tremendously enhanced by the substitution of new authors, as the former authority "standbys" stepped down or retired from our faculty. Each of the authors who continue to be selected for maintaining the character of our textbook is an authority in his or her respective area and has had considerable pedagogic and formal examination experience. One dramatic recent example of the changes in author replacement just came about with our forthcoming 17th edition. When I invited Dr. Peter Goldblatt to participate in the authorship of the pathology chapter of the textbook, his answer was "what goes around, comes around." You see, Dr. Goldblatt's father, Dr. Harry Goldblatt, a major contributor to the history of hypertensive disease, was the first author of the pathology chapter in 1931. What a satisfying experience for me personally. Other less human changes in our format came with the establishment of two soft cover volumes, the current basic and clinical sciences review volumes, replacing the single volume text of earlier years. Soon, a third supplementary volume concerned with questions and answers for the basic science volume appeared. Accompanying these more obvious changes was the constant updating of the knowledge base of each of the chapters, and this continues on into the present 17th edition.

And now we have introduced another major innovation in our presentation of the basic and clinical sciences reviews. This change is evidenced by the concurrent introduction of four volumes during this year representing four important chapters presented in the parent textbook: behavioral sciences, internal medicine, surgery, and psychiatry and behavioral medicine. Additional volumes, concerned with each of the other chapters of the parent textbook, will be published in subsequent years along with the 17th edition of *Rypins' Basic Sciences Review, Rypins' Clinical Sciences Review,* and the *Questions and Answers* third volume. These volumes are written to be used separately from the parent textbook. Each not only will contain the material published in their respective chapters of the textbook, but will be considerably "fleshed out" in the discussions, tables, figures, and questions and answers. Thus, we hope that the *Rypins' Intensive Reviews* series will serve as an important supplement to the overall review process and that it will also provide a study guide for those already in practice in preparing for specific specialty board certification and recertification examinations.

Therefore, with continued confidence and excitement, I am pleased to present these innovations in review experience for your consideration. As in the past, I look forward to learning of your comments and suggestions. In doing so, we continue to look forward to our continued growth and acceptance of the *Rypins'* review experience.

Edward D. Frohlich, MD, MACP, FACC

Series Acknowledgments

In no other writing experience is one more dependent on others than in a textbook, especially a textbook that provides a broad review for the student and fellow practitioner. In this spirit, I am truly indebted to all who have contributed to our past and current understanding of the fundamental and clinical aspects related to the practice of medicine. No one individual ever provides the singular "breakthrough" so frequently attributed as such by the news media. Knowledge develops and grows as a result of continuing and exciting contributions of research from all disciplines, academic institutions, and nations. Clearly, outstanding investigators have been credited for major contributions, but those with true and understanding humility are quick to attribute the preceding input of knowledge by others to the growing body of knowledge. In this spirit, we acknowledge the long list of contributors to medicine over the generations. We also acknowledge that in no century has man so exceeded the sheer volume of these advances than in the twentieth century. Indeed, it has been said by many that the sum of new knowledge over the past 50 years has most likely exceeded all that had been contributed in the prior years.

With this spirit of more universal acknowledgment, I wish to recognize personally the interest, support, and suggestions made by my colleagues in my institution and elsewhere. I specifically refer to those people from my institution who were of particular help and are listed at the outset of the internal medicine volume. But, in addition to these colleagues, I want to express my deep appreciation to my institution and clinic for providing the opportunity and ambience to maintain and continue these academic pursuits. As I have often said, the primary mission of a school of medicine is that of education and research; the care of patients, a long secondary mission to ensure the conduct of the primary goal, has now also become a primary commitment in these more pragmatic times. In contrast, the primary mission of the major multispecialty clinics has been the care of patients, with education and research assuming secondary roles as these commitments become affordable. It is this distinction that sets the multispecialty clinic apart from other modes of medical practice.

Over and above a personal commitment and drive to assure publication of a textbook such as this is the tremendous support and loyalty of a hard-working and dedicated office staff. To this end, I am tremendously grateful and indebted to Mrs. Lillian Buffa and Mrs. Caramia Fairchild. Their long hours of unselfish work on my behalf and to satisfy their own interest in participating in this major educational effort is appreciated no end. I am personally deeply honored and thankful for their important roles in the publication of the Rypins' series.

Words of appreciation must be extended to the staff of the Lippincott–Raven Publishers. It is more than 25 years since I have become associated with this publishing house, one of the first to be established in our nation. Over these years, I have worked closely with Mr. Richard Winters, not only with the Rypins' editions but also with other textbooks. His has been a labor of commitment, interest, and full support—not only because of his responsibility to his institution, but also because of the excitement of publishing new knowledge. In recent years, we discussed at length the merits of adding the intensive review supplements to the parent textbook and together we worked out the details that have become the substance of our present "joint venture." Moreover, together we are willing to make the necessary changes to assure the intellectual success of this series. To this end, we are delighted to include a new member of our team effort, Ms. Susan Kelly. She joined our cause to ensure that the format of questions, the reference process of answers to those questions within the text itself, and the editorial process involved be natural and clear to our readers. I am grateful for each of these facets of the overall publication process.

Not the least is my everlasting love and appreciation to my family. I am particularly indebted to my parents who inculcated in me at a very early age the love of education, the respect for study and hard work, and the honor for those who share these values. In this regard, it would have been impossible for me to accomplish any of my academic pursuits without the love, inspiration, and continued support of my wife, Sherry. Not only has she maintained the personal encouragement to initiate and continue with these labors of love, but she has sustained and supported our family and home life so that these activities could be encouraged. Hopefully, these pursuits have not detracted from the development and love of our children, Margie, Bruce, and Lara. I assume that this has not occurred; we are so very proud that each is personally committed to education and research. How satisfying it is to realize that these ideals remain a familial characteristic.

Edward D. Frohlich, MD, MACP, FACC
New Orleans, Louisiana

▼

Introduction

Preparing for USMLE

In August 1991 the Federation of State Medical Boards (FSMB) and the National Board of Medical Examiners (NBME) agreed to replace their respective examinations, the FLEX and NBME, with a new examination, the United States Medical Licensing Examination (USMLE). This examination will provide a common means for evaluating all applicants for medical licensure. It appears that this development in medical licensure will at last satisfy the needs for state medical boards licensure, the national medical board licensure, and licensure examinations for foreign medical graduates. This is because the 1991 agreement provides for a composite committee that equally represents both organizations (the FSMB and NBME) as well as a jointly appointed public member and a representative of the Educational Council for Foreign Medical Graduates (ECFMG).

As indicated in the USMLE announcement, "It is expected that students who enrolled in U.S. medical schools in the fall of 1990 or later and foreign medical graduates applying for ECFMG examinations beginning in 1993 will have access only to USMLE for purposes of licensure." The phaseout of the last regular examinations for licensure was completed in December 1994.

The new USMLE is administered in three steps. Step 1 focuses on fundamental basic biomedical science concepts, with particular emphasis on "principles and mechanisms underlying disease and modes of therapy." Step 2 is related to the clinical sciences, with examination on material necessary to practice medicine in a supervised setting. Step 3 is designed to focus on "aspects of biomedical and clinical science essential for the unsupervised practice of medicine."

Today Step 1 and Step 2 examinations are set up and scored as total comprehensive objective tests in the basic sciences and clinical sciences, respectively. The format of each part is no longer subject-oriented, that is, separated into sections specifically labeled Anatomy, Pathology, Medicine, Surgery, and so forth. Subject labels are therefore missing, and in each part questions from the different fields are intermixed or integrated so that the subject origin of any individual question is not immediately apparent, although it is known by the National Board office. Therefore, if necessary, individual subject grades can be extracted.

Step 1 is a two-day written test including questions in anatomy, biochemistry, microbiology, pathology, pharmacology, physiology, and the behavioral sciences. Each subject contributes to the examination a large number of questions designed to test not only knowledge of the subject itself but also "the subtler qualities of discrimination, judgment, and reasoning." Questions in such fields as molecular biology, cell biology, and genetics are included, as are questions to test the "candidate's recognition of the similarity or dissimilarity of diseases, drugs, and physiologic, behavioral, or pathologic processes." Problems are presented in narrative, tabular, or graphic form, followed by questions designed to assess the candidate's knowledge and comprehension of the situation described.

Step 2 is also a two-day written test that includes questions in internal medicine, obstetrics and gynecology, pediatrics, preventive medicine and public health, psychiatry, and surgery. The questions, like those in Step 1, cover a broad spectrum of knowledge in each of the clinical fields. In addition to individual questions, clinical problems are presented in the form of case histories, charts, roentgenograms, photographs of gross and microscopic pathologic specimens, laboratory data, and the like, and the candidate must answer questions concerning the interpretation of the data presented and their relation to the clinical problems. The questions are "designed to explore the extent of the candidate's knowledge of clinical situation, and to test his [or her] ability to bring information from many different clinical and basic science areas to bear upon these situations."

The examinations of both Step 1 and Step 2 are scored as a whole, certification being given on the basis of performance on the entire part, without reference to disciplinary breakdown. The grade for the examination is derived from the total number of questions answered correctly, rather than from an average of the grades in the component basic science or clinical science subjects. A candidate who fails will be required to repeat the entire examination. Nevertheless, as noted above, in spite of the interdisciplinary character of the examinations, all of the traditional disciplines are represented in the test, and separate grades for each subject can be extracted and reported separately to students, to state examining boards, or to those medical schools that request them for their own educational and academic purposes.

This type of interdisciplinary examination and the method of scoring the entire test as a unit have definite advantages, especially in view of the changing curricula in medical schools. The former type of rigid, almost standardized, curriculum, with its emphasis on specific subjects and a specified number of hours in each, has been replaced by a more liberal, open-ended curriculum, permitting emphasis in one or more fields and corresponding deemphasis in others. The result has been rather wide variations in the totality of education in different medical schools. Thus, the scoring of these tests as a whole permits accommodation to this variability in the curricula of different schools. Within the total score, weakness in one subject that has received relatively little emphasis in a given school may be balanced by strength in other subjects.

The rationale for this type of comprehensive examination as replacement for the traditional department-oriented examination in the basic sciences and the clinical sciences is given in the National Board Examiner:

The student, as he [or she] confronts these examinations, must abandon the idea of "thinking like a physiologist" in answering a question labeled "physiology" or "thinking like a surgeon" in answering a question labeled "surgery." The one question may have been written by a biochemist or a pharmacologist; the other question may have been written by an internist or a pediatrician. The pattern of these examinations will direct the student to thinking more broadly of the basic sciences in Step 1 and to thinking of patients and their problems in Step 2.

Until a few years ago, the Part I examination could not be taken until the work of the second year in medical school had been completed, and the Part II test was given only to students who had completed the major part of the fourth year. Now students, if they feel they are ready, may be admitted to any regularly scheduled Step 1 or Step 2 examination during any year of their medical course without prerequisite completion of specified courses or chronologic periods of study. Thus, emphasis is placed on the acquisition of knowledge and competence rather than the completion of predetermined periods.

Candidates are eligible for Step 3 after they have passed Steps 1 and 2, have received the M.D. degree from an approved medical school in the United States or Canada, and subsequent to the receipt of the M.D. degree, have served at least six months in an approved hospital internship or residency. Under certain circumstances, consideration may be given to other types of graduate training provided they meet with the approval of the National Board. After passing the Step 3 examination, candidates will receive their Diplomas as of the date of the satisfactory completion of an internship or residency program. If candidates have completed the approved hospital training prior to completion of Step 3, they will receive certification as of the date of the successful completion of Step 3.

The Step 3 examination, as noted above, is an objective test of general clinical competence. It occupies one full day and is divided into two sections, the first of which is a multiple-choice examination that relates to the interpretation of clinical data presented primarily in pictorial form, such as pictures of patients, gross and microscopic lesions, electrocardiograms, charts, and graphs. The second section, entitled Patient Management Problems, utilizes a programmed-testing technique designed to measure the candidate's clinical judgment in the management of patients. This technique simulates clinical situations in which the physician is faced with the problems of patient management presented in a sequential programmed pattern. A set of some four to six problems is related to each of a series of patients. In the scoring of this section, candidates are given credit for correct choices; they are penalized for errors of commission (selection of procedures that are unnecessary or are contraindicated) and for errors of omission (failure to select indicated procedures).

All parts of the National Board examinations are given in many centers, usually in medical schools, in nearly every large city in the United States as well as in a few cities in Canada, Puerto Rico, and the Canal Zone. In some cities, such as New York, Chicago, and Baltimore, the examination may be given in more than one center.

The examinations of the National Board have become recognized as the most comprehensive test of knowledge of the medical sciences and their clinical application produced in this country.

THE NATIONAL BOARD OF MEDICAL EXAMINERS

For years the National Board examinations have served as an index of the medical education of the period and have strongly influenced higher educational standards in each of the medical sciences. The Diploma of the National Board is accepted by 47 state licensing authorities, the District of Columbia, and the Commonwealth of Puerto Rico in lieu of the examination usually required for licensure and is recognized in the American Medical Directory by the letters DNB following the name of the physician holding National Board certification.

The National Board of Medical Examiners has been a leader in developing new and more reliable techniques of testing, not only for knowledge in all medical fields but also for clinical competence and fitness to practice. In recent years, too, a number of medical schools, several specialty certifying boards, professional medical societies organized to encourage their members to keep abreast of progress in medicine, and other professional qualifying agencies have called upon the National Board's professional staff for advice or for the actual preparation of tests to be employed in evaluating medical knowledge, effectiveness of teaching, and professional competence in certain medical fields. In all cases, advantage has been taken of the validity and effectiveness of the objective, multiple-choice type of examination, a technique the National Board has played an important role in bringing to its present state of perfection and discriminatory effectiveness.

Objective examinations permit a large number of questions to be asked, and approximately 150 to 180 questions can be answered in a $2\frac{1}{2}$-hour period. Because the answer sheets are scored by machine, the grading can be accomplished rapidly, accurately, and impartially. It is completely unbiased and based on percentile ranking. Of long-range significance is the facility with which the total test and individual questions can be subjected to thorough and rapid statistical analyses, thus providing a sound basis for comparative studies of medical school teaching and for continuing improvement in the quality of the test itself.

QUESTIONS

Over the years, many different forms of objective questions have been devised to test not only medical knowledge but also those subtler qualities of discrimination, judgment, and reasoning. Certain types of questions may test an individual's recognition of the similarity or dissimilarity of diseases, drugs, and physiologic or pathologic processes. Other questions test judgment as to cause and effect or the lack of causal relationships. Case histories or patient problems are used to simulate the experience of a physician confronted with a diagnostic problem; a series of questions then tests the individual's understanding of related aspects of the case, such as signs and symptoms, associated laboratory findings, treatment, complications, and prognosis. Case-history questions are set up purposely to place emphasis on correct diagnosis within a context comparable with the experience of actual practice.

It is apparent from recent certification and board examinations that the examiners are devoting more attention in their construction of questions to more practical means of testing basic and clinical knowledge. This greater realism in testing relates to an increasingly interdisciplinary approach toward fundamental material and to the direct relevance accorded practical clinical problems. These more recent approaches to questions have been incorporated into this review series.

Of course, the new approaches to testing add to the difficulty experienced by the student or physician preparing for board or certification examinations. With this in mind, the author of this review is acutely aware not only of the interrelationships of fundamental information within the basic science disciplines and their clinical implications but also of the necessity to present this material clearly and concisely despite its complexity. For this reason, the questions are devised to test knowledge of specific material within the text and identify areas for more intensive study, if necessary. Also, those preparing for examinations must be aware of the interdisciplinary nature of fundamental clinical material, the common multifactorial characteristics of disease mechanisms, and the necessity to shift back and forth from one discipline to another in order to appreciate the less than clear-cut nature separating the pedagogic disciplines.

The different types of questions that may be used on examinations include the completion-type question, where the individual must select one best answer among a number of possible choices, most often five, although there may be three or four; the completion-type question in the negative form, where all but one of the choices is correct and words such as *except* or *least* appear in the question; the true-false type of question, which tests an understanding of cause and effect in relationship to medicine; the multiple true-false type, in which the question may have one, several, or all correct choices; one matching-type question, which tests association and relatedness and uses four choices, two of which use the word, *both* or *neither;* another matching-type question that uses anywhere from three to twenty-six choices and may have more than one correct answer; and, as noted above, the patient-oriented question, which is written around a case and may have several questions included as a group or set.

Many of these question types may be used in course or practice exams; however, at this time the most commonly used types of questions on the USMLE exams are the completion-type question (one best answer), the completion-type negative form, and the multiple matching-type question, designating specifically how many choices are correct. Often included within the questions are graphic elements such as diagrams, charts, graphs, electrocardiograms, roentgenograms, or photomicrographs to elicit knowledge of structure, function, the course of a clinical situation, or a statistical tabulation. Questions then may be asked in relation to designated elements of the same. As noted above, case histories or patient-oriented questions are more frequently used on these examinations, requiring the individual to use more analytic abilities and less memorization-type data.

For further detailed information concerning developments in the evolution of the examination process for medical licensure (for graduates of both U.S. and foreign medical schools), those interested should contact the National Board of Medical Examiners at 3750 Market Street, Philadelphia, PA 19104, USA; telephone number 215–590–9500.

FIVE POINTS TO REMEMBER

In order for the candidate to maximize chances for passing these examinations, a few common sense strategies or guidelines should be kept in mind.

First, it is imperative to prepare thoroughly for the examination. Know well the types of questions to be presented and the pedagogic areas of particular weakness, and devote more preparatory study time to these areas of weakness. Do not use too much time restudying areas in which there is a feeling of great confidence and do not leave unexplored those areas in which there is less confidence. Finally, be well rested before the test and, if possible, avoid traveling to the city of testing that morning or late the evening before.

Second, know well the format of the examination and the instructions before becoming immersed in the challenge at hand. This information can be obtained from many published texts and brochures or directly from the testing service (National Board of Medical Examiners, 3750 Market Street, Philadelphia, PA 19104; telephone 215–590–9500). In addition, many available texts and self-assessment types of examination are valuable for practice.

Third, know well the overall time allotted for the examination and its components and the scope of the test to be faced. These may be learned by a rapid review of the examination itself. Then, proceed with the test at a careful, deliberate, and steady pace without spending an inordinate amount of time on any single question. For example, certain questions such as the "one best answer" probably should be allotted 1 to 1½ minutes each. The "matching" type of question should be allotted a similar amount of time.

Fourth, if a question is particularly disturbing, note appropriately the question (put a mark on the question sheet) and return to this point later. Don't compromise yourself by so concentrating on a likely "loser" that several "winners" are eliminated because of inadequate time. One way to save this time on a particular "stickler" is to play your initial choice; your chances of a correct answer are always best with your first impression. If there is no initial choice, reread the question.

Fifth, allow adequate time to review answers, to return to the questions that were unanswered and "flagged" for later attention, and check every nth (e.g., 20th) question to make certain that the answers are appropriate and that you did not inadvertently skip a question in the booklet or answer on the sheet (this can happen easily under these stressful circumstances).

There is nothing magical about these five points. They are simple and just make common sense. If you have prepared well, have gotten a good night's sleep, have eaten a good breakfast, and follow the preceding five points, the chances are that you will not have to return for a second go-around.

Edward D. Frohlich, MD, MACP, FACC

▼ Contents

CONTENTS

CONTENTS

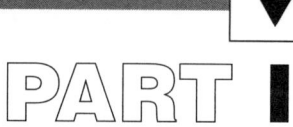

PART I

Basic Considerations

Chapter 1

Shock

Shock is a clinical syndrome that results from tissue perfusion inadequate to maintain normal metabolic and nutritional activities. Although direct histotoxic factors may play a role in the development of shock, the common denominator in all forms of shock is **reduced blood flow** to vital organs. In the clinical setting, when confronted with a patient in shock, its origin may not be readily apparent. However, because shock may rapidly progress to multisystem organ failure and death, empiric treatment is initiated while a specific cause is elucidated. The term shock describes a generalized dysfunction of the normal cardiovascular homeostatic mechanisms.

TYPES OF SHOCK

Shock can be classified into four types, according to etiology: cardiogenic, vasogenic, neurogenic, and hypovolemic (Table 1-1). In each type of shock, inadequate oxygen delivery is a common feature.

Cardiogenic Shock

Cardiogenic shock is circulatory failure caused by **failure of the heart to serve as an adequate pump**. Examples include myocardial infarction, arrhythmias, and myocardial depression. Patients demonstrate cold, clammy, cyanotic skin; urine flow is less than 20 mL/hr; and altered mental status is frequently seen. The goals of treatment should be to maintain end-organ perfusion and cardiac viability by maximizing myocardial oxygen supply while simultaneously minimizing myocardial oxygen demand.

Vasogenic Shock

Vasogenic shock is circulatory failure associated with a **decrease in peripheral vascular resistance and an increase in central capaci-**

TABLE 1-1.

Types of Shock

	Features		
Type	**Skin**	**Heart Rate**	**Blood Pressure**
Hypovolemic	Cold and clammy	Elevated	Decreased
Neurogenic	Warm, flushed	Decreased	Decreased
Cardiogenic	Cold, clammy, and cyanotic	Normal to elevated	Decreased
Vasogenic/septic			
Early	Warm and moist	Elevated	Normal
Late	Cool and clammy	Increased	Decreased

---

tance. Septic shock and shock associated with multiple organ failure are primarily examples of this type of shock.

Patients with **septic shock** usually present with hypotension, warm moist skin, mental status changes, and respiratory alkalosis. Hemodynamic monitoring frequently reveals a high cardiac output early in the course of septic shock (hyperdynamic state). In 25% of patients, however, a low cardiac output and high peripheral vascular resistance are present and consistent with a hypodynamic state. This latter group of patients is indistinguishable from patients with hypovolemic shock. These two presentations most likely represent a continuum of the same pathophysiology. The hypodynamic state is often seen late in the course when therapy has failed. The **mortality rates** from septic shock remain in the **50% to 70%** range. Fundamental features of therapy remain adequate surgical drainage of the septic focus, volume resuscitation, and appropriate antibiotic therapy.

Neurogenic Shock

Neurogenic shock follows a central **failure of the autonomic nervous system to maintain peripheral vascular resistance**. Examples are hypotension seen in spinal anesthesia or a high transection of the spinal cord. Blood pressure is often low, but in contrast to other forms of shock, it is associated with **bradycardia**. In addition, the patient has warm, dry, or even flushed skin. The goal of management is to balance volume expansion with the risk of vasopressor administration.

Hypovolemic Shock

The most common etiology of shock in surgical patients is hypovolemia. This follows a **loss of intravascular volume**—whole blood, plasma, extracellular fluid, or a combination of these. Resuscitation is achieved by replacement of intravascular volume and arrest of the source of intravascular fluid loss. Frequently, the patient is placed in the Trendelenburg position to increase central venous pressure and arterial pressure. However, in one study, the Trendelenburg position was found to have no consistent effect on venous return in healthy or hypotensive patients, and cerebral perfusion and pulmonary function may be compromised in patients who are placed in this position. Military antishock trousers (MAST) and pneumatic antishock garments (PASG) have also been shown not to alter outcome in trauma patients. Both techniques are often used, and many think they are effective.

In most intensive care units, invasive monitors are used to assess resuscitative efforts. The Swan-Ganz catheter placed in the pulmonary artery monitors cardiac output and pulmonary artery pressures (including pulmonary artery wedge pressure and central venous pressure). It is of considerable importance in providing the basis for the appropriate volume of fluid administration. Additionally, some catheters continuously monitor oxygen saturation in the pulmonary artery (mixed venous oxygen saturation), allowing for the calculation of oxygen consumption.

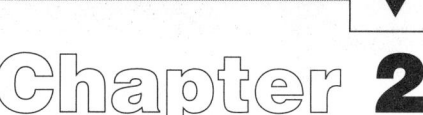

Chapter 2

Fluids and Electrolytes

MANAGING FLUID AND ELECTROLYTE BALANCE

Fluid and electrolyte management is an integral part of the care of surgical patients and may be a critical factor for many patients. Many diseases, injuries, and operative traumas have a great impact on the physiology of fluids and electrolytes, far greater than simple lack of alimentation. A prerequisite to the understanding of fluid and electrolyte management is knowledge of the extent and composition of the various body fluid compartments.

Total body water constitutes between 50% and 70% of total body weight; the average normal value is 60% of body weight for young adult men and 50% for young adult women. Fat contains less water; therefore, an obese patient has less body water than a lean patient. Total body water also decreases with age. Total body water is divided into three functional compartments (Fig. 2-1). The fluid within the body's diverse cell population, **intracellular water**, represents 60% to 70% of total body water, or 30% to 40% of total body weight. The **extracellular water** represents approximately 25% to 35% of total body water, or 20% of total body weight; this compartment is subdivided into the **intravascular fluid**, or plasma (5% of total body weight), and the **interstitial fluid** (15% of total body weight). Compositions of these fluids are shown in Figure 2-2.

Relevant to the discussion of the complicated interactions between the various body fluid compartments is the definition of commonly used terms: (1) the number of particles per unit volume (millimoles per liter; mmol/L); (2) the number of electrical charges per unit volume (milliequivalents per liter; mEq/L); and (3) the number of osmotically active particles per unit volume (milliosmoles per liter; mOsm/L). A mole of a substance is the molecular weight of that substance in grams, and a millimole is expressed in milligrams (e.g., a millimole of NaCl is 58 mg). This expression, however, provides no direct information about the number of electrical charges or osmotically active particles that a substance carries. A milliequivalent of an ion is its atomic weight expressed in milligrams divided by valence; in the case of univalent ions, a milliequivalent is the same as a millimole. In the case of divalent ions, such as calcium or magnesium, a millimole equals 2 mEq.

Rypins' Intensive Reviews: Surgery, by Ravi S. Chari and David C. Sabiston, Jr. Lippincott–Raven Publishers, Philadelphia © 1996.

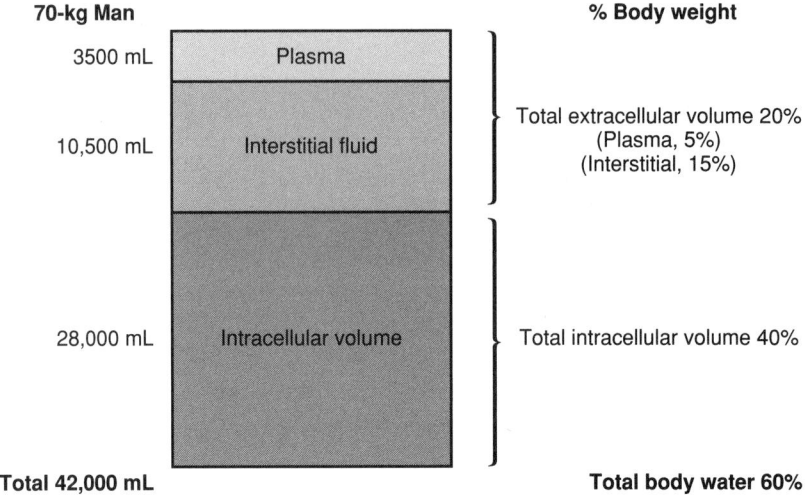

Figure 2-1.
Functional compartments of body fluids.

When **osmotic pressure** of a solution is considered, it is more descriptive to use the term **milliosmole**. This term refers to the actual number of osmotically active particles present in solution, but it is not dependent on chemical combining capacities of the substances. Therefore, 1 mmol NaCl dissociates in solution to sodium and chloride, contributing 2 mOsm; conversely, 1 mmol of an un-ionized substance, such as glucose, is equal to 1 mOsm of the substance.

The differences in ionic composition between intracellular and extracellular fluid are maintained by the cell wall, which functions

	154 mEq/L		154 mEq/L		153 mEq/L		153 mEq/L		200 mEq/L		200 mEq/L
	Cations		**Anions**		**Cations**		**Anions**		**Cations**		**Anions**
	Na^+ 142		Cl^- 103		Na^+ 144		Cl^- 114		K^+ 150		HPO_4^{3-} ⎱150 SO_4^{2-} ⎰
			HCO_3^- 27				HCO_3^- 30				
			SO_4^{2-} ⎱3 PO_4^{3-} ⎰		K^+ 4		SO_4^{2-} ⎱3 PO_4^{3-} ⎰				HCO_3^- 10
	K^+ 4		Organic acids 5		Ca^{2+} 3		Organic acids 5		Mg^{2+} 40		Protein 40
	Ca^{2+} 5		Protein 16		Mg^{2+} 2		Protein 1		Na^+ 10		
	Mg^{2+} 3										
	Plasma				**Interstitial fluid**				**Intracellular fluid**		

Figure 2-2.
Chemical composition of body fluid compartments.

as a semipermeable membrane. The total number of osmotically active particles is 290 to 310 mOsm in each compartment. Although the osmotic pressure of a fluid is the sum of the partial pressures contributed by each of the solutes in that solution, the **effective osmotic pressure** is dependent on those substances that fail to pass through the pores of the semipermeable membrane. The dissolved proteins in the plasma, therefore, are primarily responsible for the effective osmotic pressure between the plasma and the interstitial fluid. This is frequently referred to as the **colloid oncotic pressure**. Because the cell membranes are completely permeable to water, the effective oncotic pressures between the two compartments are considered equal; any condition that alters the effective oncotic pressure in either compartment results in the redistribution of water between the compartments.

The disorders of fluid balance may be classified in three general categories: disturbances of volume, concentration, and composition.

If an isotonic salt solution is added or lost from the body, there is a change in **volume**. The acute loss of an isotonic extracellular solution, such as intestinal juice, is followed by a significant decrease in the extracellular fluid volume and little, if any, change in the intracellular fluid volume. Fluid will not be transferred from the interstitial space to refill the extracellular space as long as the osmolality remains the same in the two compartments. If water alone is added to or lost from the extracellular space, the **concentration** of osmotically active particles changes. Sodium ions represent the majority of osmotically active particles in the extracellular space. The concentration of most other ions within the extracellular fluid compartment can be altered without a significant change in the number of osmotically active particles, thus producing only a **compositional** change.

An internal loss of extracellular fluid into a nonfunctional space (third space)—such as sequestration of isotonic fluid in a burn, peritonitis, ascites, or muscle trauma—is termed a **distributional** change. This transfer or functional loss of extracellular fluid internally may be extracellular (as in peritonitis) or intracellular (as in hemorrhagic shock). In any event, all distributional shifts or losses cause a contraction of the functional extracellular space.

DISORDERS ASSOCIATED WITH FLUID AND ELECTROLYTE BALANCE

Hyponatremia

Acute symptomatic hyponatremia clinically is characterized by central nervous system (CNS) signs of **increased intracranial pressure** and tissue signs of **excessive intracellular water**. There are no cardiovascular signs per se. The hypertension is induced by the rise in intracranial pressure, since the blood pressure returns to normal after correction of the hyponatremia. Many hyponatremic states are asymptomatic until the sodium level falls below 120 mEq/L. One important exception is the patient with increased cerebrospinal pressure, such as following head injury in which mild hyponatremia may be deleterious or even fatal. Also of importance with severe hyponatremia is the relatively rapid development of oliguric renal failure, which may be irreversible if therapy is delayed. Osmolality may increase, decrease, or remain unchanged in hyponatremia.

A 5% sodium chloride solution is used for immediate correction of severe symptomatic hyponatremia. The sodium deficit can be calculated by multiplying the deficit of serum sodium below normal (in mEq/L) by the liters of total body water. Note that the estimate is based on total body water, since the effective osmotic pressure in the extracellular compartment cannot be increased without increasing this fraction proportionally in the intracellular compartment. Generally, only a portion of the total deficit is replaced initially to relieve acute symptoms.

Further correction is facilitated when renal function is restored by correction of the volume deficit. Of importance, central pontine and extrapontine myelinolysis may occur with rapid correction of hyponatremia and may cause irreversible CNS damage or death. It is recommended, therefore, that the serum sodium level be increased by no more than 12 mEq/L during the first 24 hours, and even less during each subsequent 24-hour period.

Hypernatremia

CNS restlessness and delirium, as well as tissue signs (decreased saliva, dry sticky mucous membranes), characterize symptomatic hypernatremia. This is the only state in which dry, sticky mucous membranes are characteristic. This sign does not occur with extracellular volume deficit alone and usually is only an indication that the patient is breathing through the mouth. Body temperature is generally elevated and may approach a lethal level. Osmolality always increases in hypernatremia.

For the correction of severe, symptomatic hypernatremia with an associated volume deficit, D_5W may be infused slowly until symptoms are relieved. If extracellular osmolality is reduced too rapidly, however, convulsions and coma may result as water shifts into brain cells. For this reason, correction of hypernatremia is best accomplished with administration of half-strength balanced saline solution. In the absence of a significant volume deficit, water should be administered cautiously because hypervolemia may result.

Hyperkalemia

The signs of significant hyperkalemia are limited to cardiovascular and gastrointestinal symptoms. The gastrointestinal symptoms include nausea and vomiting, intermittent intestinal colic, and diarrhea. The cardiovascular symptoms apparent in the electrocardiogram are initially peaked T waves, widened QRS complexes, and depressed S-T segments. Disappearance of the T waves, heart block, and diastolic cardiac arrest may develop with increasing levels of potassium.

Treatment is directed at immediate cessation of exogenous potassium administration, measures to stabilize the myocardium, and maneuvers to decrease serum potassium. Temporary suppression of the myocardium effects of a sudden rapid rise in potassium can be accomplished by the intravenous administration of 1 g of 10% calcium gluconate under ECG monitoring. Serum potassium levels may be decreased transiently by administration of bicarbonate (45 mEq) and glucose with insulin (1000 mL $D_{10}W$ with 20 units regular insulin); both cause an intracellular shift of potassium ions. These maneuvers are temporary and allow time for definitive removal of excess potassium by cation-exchange resins, peritoneal dialysis, or hemodialysis.

Hypokalemia

A more common problem in the surgical patient is hypokalemia, which can occur as a result of (1) excessive renal excretion, (2) movement of potassium into cells, (3) prolonged administration of potassium-free parenteral fluids with continued obligatory loss of potassium, (4) parenteral nutrition with inadequate potassium administration, and (5) loss of gastrointestinal secretions (vomiting and diarrhea).

The signs of potassium deficit are related to failure of normal contractility of skeletal, smooth, and cardiac muscle and include weakness that may progress to flaccid paralysis, diminished to absent tendon reflexes, and paralytic ileus. Sensitivity to digitalis with cardiac arrhythmias and electrocardiographic signs of low voltage, flattening of T waves, and depression of S-T segments are characteristic.

The treatment of hypokalemia involves, first, prevention of this state. In replacement, no more than 40 mEq should be added to 1 L, and no more than 40 mEq should be administered in 1 hour (unless there is ECG monitoring). Generally, potassium should be given to an oliguric patient during the first 24 hours following severe surgical stress or trauma.

Acid-Base Balance

The pH (the negative logarithm of the hydrogen ion concentration) of the body fluids is normally maintained within narrow limits despite the rather large load of acid produced endogenously as a byproduct of body metabolism. The acids are neutralized efficiently by several buffer systems and subsequently are excreted by the lungs and kidneys. The important buffers include proteins and phosphates (which play a primary role in maintaining intracellular pH) and the bicarbonate-carbonic acid system (which operates principally in the extracellular fluid space). Proteins have only a minor influence in the extracellular fluid space, but hemoglobin is of prime significance as a buffer in the red blood cells.

A buffer system consists of a weak acid or base and the salt of that acid or base. The buffering effect results from the formation of an amount of weak acid or base equivalent to the amount of strong acid or base added to the system. The resultant pH change is considerably less than it would be if the substance were added to water alone. Thus, inorganic acids (HCl, H_2SO_4, H_3PO_4) and organic acids (lactic, pyruvic, keto) combine with base bicarbonate, producing the sodium salt and carbonic acid:

$$HCl + NaHCO_3 \rightarrow NACl + H_2CO_3 \rightarrow H_2O + CO_2$$

The carbonic acid formed is excreted via the lungs as CO_2. The inorganic ions are excreted via the kidneys with hydrogen or as ammonia salts. The organic ions are generally metabolized as the underlying disorder is corrected.

The four types of acid-base disturbances are listed in Table 2-1. Each disorder consists of a primary defect and a compensation. Primary respiratory abnormalities are compensated by renal mechanisms and vice versa. Knowledge of the pH, bicarbonate concentrate, and P_{CO_2} allows an accurate diagnosis of most acid-base abnormalities.

Metabolic Acidosis

Metabolic acidosis follows the retention or production of acids (diabetic ketoacidosis, lactic acidosis, azotemia) or the loss of bicarbonate-rich fluid (diarrhea, pancreatic or small bowel fistula). Initial compensation is pulmonary. Generally, in compensated metabolic acidosis, the decrease in bicarbonate (in mEq/L) should equal the decrease in P_{CO_2} (in mm Hg).

The causes of metabolic acidosis can be divided into two manageable groups by determining the anion gap. This is calculated

TABLE 2-1.

Four Types of Acid-Base Disturbances

Type	Primary Defect	Compensation
Respiratory alkalosis	Decreased P_{CO_2}	Renal: decreased $[HCO_3^-]$
Metabolic alkalosis	Increased $[HCO_3^-]$	Respiratory: increased P_{CO_2}
Respiratory acidosis	Increased P_{CO_2}	Renal: increased $[HCO_3^-]$
Metabolic acidosis	Decreased $[HCO_3^-]$	Respiratory: decreased P_{CO_2}

simply by subtracting the sum of the bicarbonate and chloride concentrations from the sodium concentration. The normal value is 10 to 15 mEq/L. The anion gap represents the unmeasured anions as sulfate, phosphate, lactate, and other organic anions (Fig. 2-3). If acidosis is due to a **loss of bicarbonate** or a **gain of chloride**, the anion gap is normal. Conversely, if the acidosis is due to the increased production of an organic acid, or the retention of a sulfuric or phosphoric acid (as in renal failure), then the anion gap increases. In pure anion gap metabolic acidosis, the increase in anion gap above the normal value (approximately 12 mEq/L) should equal the decrease in bicarbonate (Table 2-2).

The treatment of metabolic acidosis is directed toward the correction of the underlying disorder when possible. The most common cause of metabolic acidosis in surgical patients is acute circulatory failure with accumulation of lactic acid. Intravenous administration of bicarbonate is reserved for the treatment of severe metabolic acidosis (pH less than 7.20), when partial correction of pH may be essential to restore myocardial function.

Metabolic Alkalosis

Metabolic alkalosis follows loss of fixed acids or gain of bicarbonate and is aggravated by an existing potassium deficit. Respiratory compensation is minimal in most patients. The causes of metabolic alkalosis can be divided into two major groups: chloride responsive (urine chloride less than 10 to 20 mEq/L) and **chloride resistant** (urine chloride more than 20 mEq/L) (Table 2-3). States of chloride-resistant metabolic alkalosis are associated with normal to slightly increased extracellular fluid volume. The treatment is directed toward the underlying cause of fluid retention.

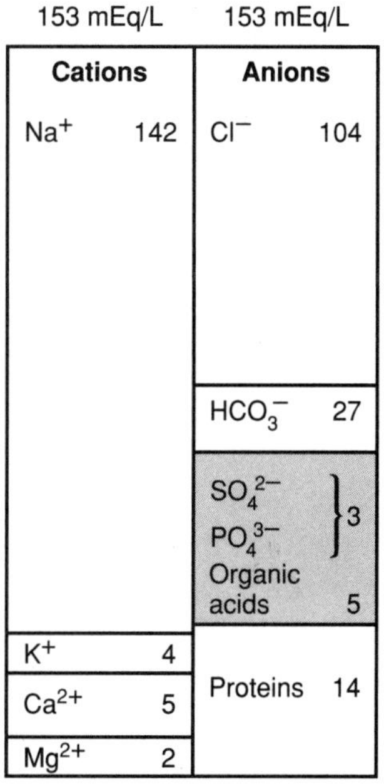

Figure 2-3.
The anion gap.

TABLE 2-2.
Causes of Metabolic Acidosis

Causes	Mechanisms
Nonanion Gap	
Diarrhea, small bowel fistula, ureterosigmoidostomy	Loss of HCO_3^-
Proximal renal tubular acidosis	Decreased tubular reabsorption of HCO_3^-
Distal renal tubular acidosis	Decreased acid excretion
Administration of NH_4Cl, HCl	Increased acid load
"Dilutional" acidosis	Volume expansion with HCO_3^- free fluids
Anion Gap	
Shock	Increased lactic acid
Diabetes, starvation, alcohol intoxication	Increased ketoacids
Uremia (renal failure)	Retention of sulfuric and phosphoric acids
Ingestion of: methanol ethylene glycol aspirin	Conversion to: formic acid oxalic acid salicylic acid

Chloride-responsive types of metabolic alkalosis are considerably more common and are often associated with **extracellular volume deficits** (especially following diuretic therapy). In addition to volume replacement, the provision of an adequate amount of potassium is a prerequisite to restoration of normal acid-base and potassium equilibrium. It should be emphasized that alkalemic patients are invariably hypokalemic, and potassium depletion itself may induce metabolic acidosis.

The prototype for chloride-responsive, hypochloremic, hypokalemic metabolic alkalosis is that which occurs from persistent vomiting or prolonged nasogastric suction in the presence of an obstructed pylorus. There is loss of high chloride and hydrogen concentrations relative to sodium, and there is extravascular volume depletion. The latter stimulates sodium ion reabsorption in the distal renal tubules in exchange for hydrogen and potassium ions. Thus, there is continued loss of potassium (from vomiting and renal exchange), requiring hydrogen to be exchanged for sodium—this worsens the alkalemia (the urine, therefore, can be paradoxically acetic).

Treatment involves the replacement of extracellular fluid volume deficit with isotonic saline solution. Potassium can be added after good urinary output has been established.

TABLE 2-3.

Metabolic Alkalosis

Chloride Responsive (Urine Cl⁻ < 10–20 mEq/L)

Vomiting

Gastric suctioning with obstructed pylorus

Diuretics

Villous adenoma of the colon

Chloride Resistant (Urine Cl⁻ > 20 mEq/L)

Primary hyperaldosteronism

Cushing's disease

Exogenous corticosteroids

Chronic hypokalemia

Unclassified

Alkali ingestion or infusion

Respiratory Acidosis

In most instances, the underlying cause of respiratory acidosis is readily apparent by history and physical examination. Respiratory acidosis is caused by **retention of CO_2**, secondary to decreased alveolar ventilation. A number of conditions cause inadequate ventilation, including pneumonia, atelectasis, pleural effusion, and hypoventilation due to abdominal incisions. These problems are particularly serious in patients with chronic obstructive pulmonary disease (COPD).

Management of respiratory acidosis involves prompt establishment of adequate alveolar ventilation. Depending on the clinical situation, this can be accomplished with administration of analgesics, bronchodilators, or endotracheal intubation.

Respiratory Alkalosis

Hyperventilation due to apprehension, pain, hypoxemia, CNS injury, and assisted ventilation are common causes of respiratory alkalosis. Any of these conditions may cause a **decrease in P_{CO_2}** and **elevation of pH**. Severe metabolic alkalosis may cause serious impairment of both cardiovascular and cerebral functions. Another effect of alkalosis is a left-shift of the oxygen dissociation curve, which may limit the ability of hemoglobin to unload oxygen to tissues.

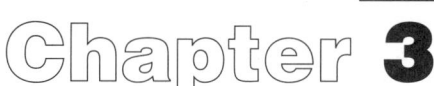

Chapter 3

Wound Healing

The process of wound healing concerns the tissue's response to injury. In humans, the wound healing response is traditionally divided into three phases: **inflammation, fibroplasia, and maturation**. The latter phases of inflammation and the early phases of fibroplasia are better described in terms of cellular events, namely stages of cell migration and proliferation. The steps overlap broadly with each other, and the process is a continuum rather than a series of discrete changes.

WOUND HEALING PROCESS

Following disruption in the tissue, the integrity of the blood vessels is disturbed, exposing the blood to collagen and subendothelial parenchyma, which is generally considered the initiating factor in wound healing. Even this initial phase is complex: blood extravasates, distorts tissue surfaces, and initiates an acute inflammatory response. Concurrently, a hemostatic response is initiated. An initial period of intense vasoconstriction follows direct vascular trauma. Platelets are activated and aggregate, and the clotting cascade is initiated. Both the kininogen and the complement cascades are activated, causing vasodilatation and an increase in capillary permeability. Injury activates local factors, which cause an orderly and predictable migration of cells into the wound. A cascade of cell activation and cytokine release ensues, which stimulates mitotic and synthetic activities of the immigrating cells. The migratory phase is initiated within hours.

An efflux of **polymorphonuclear leukocytes** from the vascular space follows rapidly, with phagocytic elimination of bacteria from the wound. Although neutrophils decrease infection, they are not essential to normal healing of sterile wounds. The second cell to make its appearance, the blood monocyte (called a macrophage after it leaves the circulation), is not only phagocytic, but is of central importance in regulating subsequent cellular activities in the healing process in the wound.

Fibroblasts migrate into the wound during the first week, and the proliferative phase of fibroplasia begins. Fibroblasts not only multiply and migrate, but they also elaborate both interstitial matrix and **collagen**. The macrophage appears to be the prime factor in regulating collagen elaboration by the fibroblasts. Initially, type III collagen is secreted in higher concentrations than type I—70% and 30%, respectively (Table 3-1). After 48 to 60 hours, the ratio of type I to type III returns to normal (90%:10%). Collagens are rich in glycine and proline, and prolines are responsible for the tight alpha helical structure. Collagen synthesis and wound healing are suppressed by decreased PO_2 in the healing tissues and by low blood flow. Additionally, vitamin C deficiency, diabetes, liver insufficiency, renal insufficiency (uremia), malignancy, and administration of corticosteroids impair wound healing. The administration of corticosteroids can be mitigated by administration of vitamin A.

Additional processes characterizing fibroplasia in the repair of wounds include wound **contraction** and **reepithelialization**. Contraction is a gradual decrease in the size of the wound caused by retraction of the mass of central granulation tissue. How a wound contracts remains unclear; however, central to contracture is the **myofibroblast**. This cell is found in granulation tissue and appears to be morphologically and physiologically an intermediate between smooth muscle and fibroblast. These cells contain both actin and myosin filaments. Skin grafting (especially full-thickness skin grafts) appears to be one of the most effective methods of controlling contraction. Within 12 hours of epidermal wounding, epithelial changes occur with loosening of cell-cell and cell-matrix contacts. Epithelial cells begin to migrate over the collagen-fibronectin wound surface. Migration into the wound occurs as a rolling sheet-type migration, whereas proliferation occurs behind the wound edge by division of stem cells.

TABLE 3-1.

Four Major Types of Collagen

Type	Tissue Distribution
I	Skin, tendon, bone, ligaments, cornea, internal organs
	Accounts for 90% of body collagen
II	Cartilage, intervertebral disk, vitreous of the eye
III	Skin, blood vessels, internal organs
IV	Basal lamina

TYPES OF SUTURES

The type of suture material used influences wound healing because all suture materials are foreign bodies. No suture material produced for clinical use is devoid of tissue reaction, although inert metals and plastics stimulate minimal response. In the face of infections, **nonabsorbable sutures** act as foreign bodies and perpetuate the infection until they are extruded or removed. **Absorbable sutures** range in times for absorption from a few days (catgut), to weeks (Dexon, Vicryl), to months (PDS, Maxon). Nonabsorbable sutures are subcategorized as monofilament or braided. **Monofilament sutures** are less conducive to infection than are multifilament sutures of the same material (Table 3-2). The selection of suture material is based on characteristics of the suture, individual preference of the surgeon, suture availability, and tissue to be sutured.

CARE OF WOUNDS

In traumatic or contaminated wounds associated with tissue destruction, wounds should be thoroughly cleaned and debrided. Primary closure may be feasible in some wounds, but the wound may be left open and allowed to heal by secondary intention or by secondary plastic procedures. The three phases of wound healing

TABLE 3-2.

Types of Sutures

Absorbable	Nonabsorbable
Natural	Monofilament
Catgut	Natural
Chromic catgut	Steel
Synthetic	Synthetic
Monofilament	Nylon
Polydiaxone (PDS)	Polypropelene
Monocryl	Braided
Maxon	Natural
Braided	Cotton
Vicryl	Silk
Dexon	Synthetic
	Dacron
	Ticron
	Nylon

previously discussed occur in the same progression whether the wound is closed primarily or left open.

Finally, cellular and matrix changes in the wound continue long after the completion of epithelialization. Wound strength increases significantly over the first 6 weeks after injury, and then only slightly over the next 2 years. It is important to note that there is **no appreciable increase in collagen content 21 days after wounding**. The clinical appearance of a scar over time, with decreasing hyperemia, reflects a decrease in vascularity and progressive organization and maturation of fibrotic tissue.

Chapter 4

Surgical Drains

Surgical drainage may be thought of as a therapeutic maneuver (i.e., to drain pus), a prophylactic maneuver, or a decompressive maneuver (i.e., to prevent fluid accumulation). Most of the basic tenets of surgical drainage were established by the end of the 19th century and, surprisingly, few scientific studies of drains or drainage have appeared since that time. Thus, many controversies persist. Today, the widespread use of prophylactic antibiotics in surgery has gradually displaced the prophylactic use of drains. There seems to be little reason to insert drains solely to prevent infection, particularly when prophylactic antibiotics are administered concurrently.

Ideally, a drain should evacuate the effluent that is to be removed, prevent damage to the surrounding tissues, prevent the introduction of infection, and be able to be removed readily. Drains are most commonly classified as open or closed suction drains. In contemporary practice, new radiographic techniques have dramatically changed the way deep fluid collections are diagnosed and managed.

OPEN DRAINS

Passive open drains, such as a Penrose drain, function mainly to **establish a tract**, or path, of least resistance **to the outside**. Like most drains, they should be led out through a separate site rather than through the primary surgical incision. They are especially useful for draining large abscess cavities in which pus is likely to accumulate in the absence of a drain.

In modern practice, there is probably no justification for the routine placement of an open drain in clean or clean-contaminated surgical wounds. Previously, it was advocated that these drains be placed in the subhepatic space following bowel anastomoses and in the perineum following abdominoperineal resections. Under such circumstances, open drainage serves merely to promote retrograde bacterial infection, retard healing, and delay recovery.

CLOSED-SUCTION DRAINS

Closed-suction drainage is most useful for **removing large volumes of relatively nonviscid fluids**, such as pancreatic or enteric secretions, bile, and urine, from deep body cavities. With the exception of chest tubes, most closed-suction drains are relatively small in diameter; thus, they are unreliable as indicators of postoperative bleeding. When compared with open drains, closed-suction drains pose less risk of retrograde bacterial infection, provided the drain is left in pace for no more than a few days. Short-term antibiotic prophylaxis can further reduce the risk.

PERCUTANEOUS, RADIOLOGICALLY GUIDED CATHETERS

The percutaneous, radiographically guided catheter of deep fluid collections is still relatively new and, with rapid changes in technology, the principles governing its use are hard to define. This technique is especially useful in the management of abdominal abscesses.

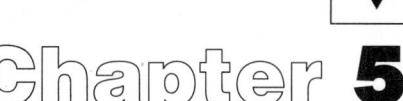

Chapter 5

Surgical Infections

Infection of surgical wounds follows bacterial contamination from either the patient's internal environment (including the skin) or from breaks in surgical technique (e.g., from the surgical team). Breaks in surgical technique are very rare. Infection of the surgical wound is complex, and the number and virulence of the microbes involved are related to many factors, including systemic diseases (e.g., diabetes mellitus), nutritional status, immunosuppression, and operative factors such as the presence of dead and devitalized tissue, hematoma, foreign bodies, and seroma formation. During the surgical procedure, the surgeon may increase the chance of infection by handling the tissue roughly and causing foci of necrosis (including tissue that has been clamped with hemostats, overusing electrocautery), using inadequate aseptic technique, failing to establish adequate hemostasis, and approximating the wound incorrectly.

Classification of Wounds

Surgical wounds have been classified to develop a better understanding of surgical infections and to form the basis of management strategies. The current scheme used to classify surgical infections is shown in Table 5-1.

Clean Wounds

In clean wounds, the only source of contamination is the patient's skin. Infection rates are less than 2%. Unless a foreign body (e.g., joint prosthesis, vascular prosthesis) is deliberately inserted or the procedure is anticipated to be of lengthy duration, no antimicrobial prophylaxis is indicated.

Clean-Contaminated Wounds

In clean-contaminated wounds, the contamination may arise from the skin and an opening in the biliary tract, gastrointestinal tract

TABLE 5-1.

Classification of Operative Wounds in Relation to Contamination and Increasing Risk of Infection

Clean

Elective, primarily closed and undrained

Nontraumatic, noninflamed, uninfected

No break in asepsis

Respiratory, alimentary, genitourinary, or oropharyngeal tracts not entered

Clean-Contaminated

Respiratory, alimentary, genitourinary or oropharyngeal entered under controlled conditions, without unusual contamination; noninfected biliary and genitourinary tracts

Mechanical drainage

Minor break in technique

Contaminated

Open, fresh, traumatic wound

Entrance of biliary and genitourinary tracts in presence of infected bile or urine

Major break in technique

Incisions in which acute nonpurulent inflammation is present

Dirty or Infected

Traumatic wound with retained devitalized tissue, foreign bodies, or fecal contamination

Perforated viscus encountered

Acute bacterial inflammation with pus encountered during operation

(including appropriately prepared large bowel), or respiratory tree. Rates of wound infection are between 3% and 4%. Prophylaxis consists of antimicrobial therapy directed against skin flora and the anticipated flora of any of the viscera that are to be opened.

Contaminated and Dirty Wounds

The final two categories of surgical infections are as described in Table 5-1. For **contaminated wounds**, infection rates are approximately 8.5%, and rates of 28% to 40% have been reported for **dirty wounds**.

Treatment

Currently, preoperative **antibiotic prophylaxis** is recommended as a single dose, 1 hour before initiation of the procedure, which assures that peak drug levels are coincident with the time of incision. Generally, postoperative antibiotics are not recommended for prophylaxis of wound infection, although many surgeons administer one or two doses postoperatively. Antibiotic prophylaxis is recommended for clean cases with implanted foreign bodies and for clean-contaminated cases. In heavily contaminated and infected wounds, treatment that is continued after the surgical procedure is no longer considered prophylactic, since the antibiotics are given for a presumed or documented infection.

Cellulitis is a spreading infection of the skin and subcutaneous tissues in which there may be evidence of cutaneous injury. It is characterized by local pain, tenderness, edema, and erythema. Usually the border between the involved and uninvolved skin is indistinct. *Streptococcus pyogenes* (Lancefield group A streptococci) is the most common organism causing cellulitis, although *Staphylococcus aureus*, *Streptococcus pneumoniae* and other streptococci, *Haemophilus influenzae*, and aerobic and anaerobic bacteria may be the cause. Extension of the infection along the course of the lymphatics is manifested by development of red streaks with local tenderness (lymphangitis). The regional lymph nodes may also become enlarged and tender.

Erysipelas

Erysipelas is a special type of cellulitis also caused by *S. pyogenes*. In contrast to cellulitis, erysipelas is characterized by a raised, sharply demarcated advancing margin.

The appropriate treatment of cellulitis consists of antibiotics, application of heat locally, adequate immobilization, and elevation. Cellulitis often subsides with appropriate therapy, but it may progress to the formation of an abscess, which requires surgical drainage.

Soft Tissue Abscess

Surgical treatment is often required for soft tissue infections, which cause tissue necrosis or an abscess.

Carbuncle

A carbuncle is a subcutaneous abscess, usually formed by a confluent infection of multiple hair follicles. *Staphylococcus* is the most frequent microorganism cultured in this clinical setting. Overlying edema may lead to the mistaken diagnosis of cellulitis, but the presence of a fluctuant mass usually leads to the correct diagnosis.

Felon

A felon is a purulent collection in the distal phalanx of the finger that causes intense pain and pressure in that compartment. Swelling may be minimal because of the fibrous bands between the skin and bone. Treatment requires incision and drainage.

Breast Abscess

Breast abscess is usually caused by *S. aureus,* but it also can be caused by gram-negative bacteria. It frequently occurs in nursing mothers. Treatment consists of incision and drainage and appropriate antibiotics.

Perirectal Abscess

Perirectal abscess begins as an infection of one of the crypt glands and then extends into the perirectal space and at times presents subcutaneously near the anus. It is caused by aerobic and anaerobic bacteria, which are normally found in the colon. Incision and drainage and antibiotic therapy are the appropriate initial treatment. Up to 50% of perirectal abscesses may cause a fistula communication with the anal crypt and may require future treatment.

NECROTIZING SOFT TISSUE INFECTIONS

Soft tissue infections that produce tissue necrosis are less common than other forms of soft tissue infections, but they are more serious because of their propensity for **extensive tissue destruction and high mortality rate**. The nomenclature for necrotizing soft tissue infections is confusing and has been based on the causative organism and tissue affected. Terms such as necrotizing fasciitis, streptococcal gangrene, gas gangrene, bacterial synergistic gangrene, clostridial myonecrosis, streptococcal myonecrosis, and Fournier's gangrene are commonly used.

Attempts to differentiate these infections clinically are based on predisposing conditions, presence of pain, toxicity, fever, presence of crepitus, appearance of the skin and subcutaneous tissues, and the presence or absence of bullae. Such classifications and clinical appearance are of little aid in the initial treatment of these infections. Bacteria seldom respect anatomic barriers; thus, necrotizing fasciitis is rarely limited to fascia and myonecrosis is rarely limited to muscle.

Most necrotizing soft tissue infections are caused by mixed aerobic and anaerobic gram-negative and gram-positive bacteria.

Clostridium species are the most common cause of the most dramatic infections with rapid progression, early toxicity, and high mortality rates. The term gas gangrene has been used to indicate clostridial infection, but the presence of gas in the tissue simply implies anaerobic metabolism (hydrogen, methane, and nitrogen by-products). Both facultative and obligate anaerobes are capable of such activity. Gas in tissues is more likely *not* to be caused by *Clostridium* species.

Necrotizing soft tissue infections must be recognized early and **treated promptly**. Diagnosis is not difficult when skin necrosis, crepitus, and bullae are present, but the clinical findings can be subtle before extensive necrosis has occurred. Mental confusion, toxicity, and failure to respond to nonsurgical therapy may be early clues to a necrotizing infection. Surgical treatment requires debridement of all necrotic tissue. Amputation may be required for myonecrosis of the extremities. Tissue should be sent for Gram's staining and culture to identify the involved organisms. The use of hyperbaric oxygen to treat all necrotizing infections is controversial. It appears to be most useful in the treatment of necrotizing infections caused by *Clostridium* species.

TETANUS

Tetanus is an infection caused by a strict anaerobe, ***Clostridium tetani***. It is found in **puncture wounds** and in wounds in which there is necrotic tissue and poor blood supply. The organisms are found in the excreta of animals, especially cows and horses. Hence, wounds contaminated by street dirt and fertilized soil are most susceptible to infection by the tetanus organism.

C. tetani is a gram-positive rod that forms a spore resembling a tennis racket. *C. tetani* produces two exotoxins—tetanospasmin and tetanolysin. Tetanolysin is cardiotoxic and causes hemolysis but is not thought to be of major clinical importance. **Tetanospasmin** released into the wound binds to peripheral neuron terminals and is transported to the central nervous system both by blood and along nerve trunks. It then enters the synapse, where it acts on the inhibitory interneurons to block neurotransmitter release, resulting in heightened reflex motor activity. By a similar mechanism, the toxin causes heightened sympathetic activity. Its action causes convulsions and spasticity in response to external stimuli. When extensor muscles of the neck and back are in spasm, a convulsive contraction with the head pulled back (*opisthotonos*) and a facial grimace (*risus sardonicus*) occur. Because the autonomic nervous system is involved, hypertension, tachycardia, and cardiac arrhythmias occur. Death occurs from asphyxia, the result of diaphragmatic spasm or exhaustion.

TABLE 5-2.

Recommendations for Tetanus Prophylaxis in Routine Wound Management

History of Tetanus Toxoid	Clean Minor Wounds		All Other Wounds	
	Td*	TIG	Td*	TIG
Unknown or <3 doses	Yes	No	Yes	Yes
>3 doses†	No	No	No‡	No

Td: tetanus-diphtheria toxoid; TIG: tetanus immune globulin.
*For children younger than 7 years, DPT (diptheria, pertusis, tetanus) or DT (diphtheria and tetanus) if pertusis vaccine contraindicated.
†If only three doses given, a fourth should be administered.
‡Yes, if older than 5 years.

Treatment

Therapy involves penicillin to eradicate the source of the toxin and **tetanus immune globulin** (TIG) to neutralize the circulating and unbound toxin. The antibody in TIG has no effect on toxin already bound to neural tissue.

Meticulous wound care is the greatest prerequisite for tetanus prophylaxis, which includes irrigation, thorough debridement of dead and devitalized tissue, and removal of foreign bodies. A guide to the use of active and passive immunization prophylaxis following the recommendations of the United States Public Health Service Committee on Immunization Practices is shown in Table 5-2. Basic immunization with adsorbed toxoid requires three injections: an initial injection is given, followed by the second 4 to 6 weeks later, and the third is given 6 to 12 months later.

RABIES

In 1991, three patients in the United States died of rabies disease. Approximately 10,000 people receive postexposure prophylaxis for rabies annually. The circumstances surrounding the bite often provide clues as to whether a vaccine is indicated, such as an unprovoked attack by a domestic animal or exposure to dogs outside the United States. It is the latter category that accounts for more than 50% of cases of rabies in the United States. Bites on the hands and face carry the highest risk. Contact with blood, urine, or feces of a rabid animal does not constitute exposure; therefore, prophylaxis is not indicated.

TABLE 5-3.

Rabies Postexposure Prophylaxis Guide

Animal Type	Postexposure Prophylaxis Recommendations
Dogs and cats	No prophylaxis until animal develops symptoms*
Skunks, raccoons, bats, foxes, and most other carnivores	Immediate vaccinations
Livestock, rodents, and logomorphs (rabbits and hares)	Consult public health officials; bites of squirrels, hamsters, guinea pigs, gerbils, chipmunks, rats, mice, rodents, rabbits, and hares almost never require treatment

*During a 10-day holding period, begin treatment with HRIG and HDCV or RVA at first sign in a dog or cat that has bitten someone. The symptomatic animal should be killed immediately and tested.

Treatment

The decision to administer vaccine for prophylaxis is based on the severity of the wound and the availability of the animal for observation and autopsy purposes to substantiate the diagnosis of rabies (Table 5-3).

Postexposure prophylaxis in addition to local wound care consists of human rabies immune globulin (HRIG) and vaccine. Currently, two **rabies vaccines** are available: human diploid cell rabies vaccine (**HDCV**) or rabies vaccine adsorbed (**RVA**). Either is administered in conjunction with HRIG at the beginning of postexposure prophylaxis. The first dose is given as soon as possible after exposure. Additional doses are given on days 3, 7, 14, and 28 after the initial injection.

For adults, the vaccine should be given in the deltoid area; for children, the anterolateral aspect of the thigh is also acceptable. The gluteal region should never be used for injection of RVA or HDCV, because it results in lower neutralizing antibody titers. HRIG is administered only once (20 IU/kg) and is injected in the gluteal region.

SNAKEBITES

In North America, all poisonous snakes of medical importance are members of the *Crotalidae* family (pit vipers), with the exception of the coral snake (*Elapidae* family) (Fig. 5-1). The pit vipers include the rattlesnake, cottonmouth, water moccasin, and copperhead. **Rattlesnake bites** account for approximately 70% of all deaths due to snakebites. Death from a copperhead bite is extremely rare. The

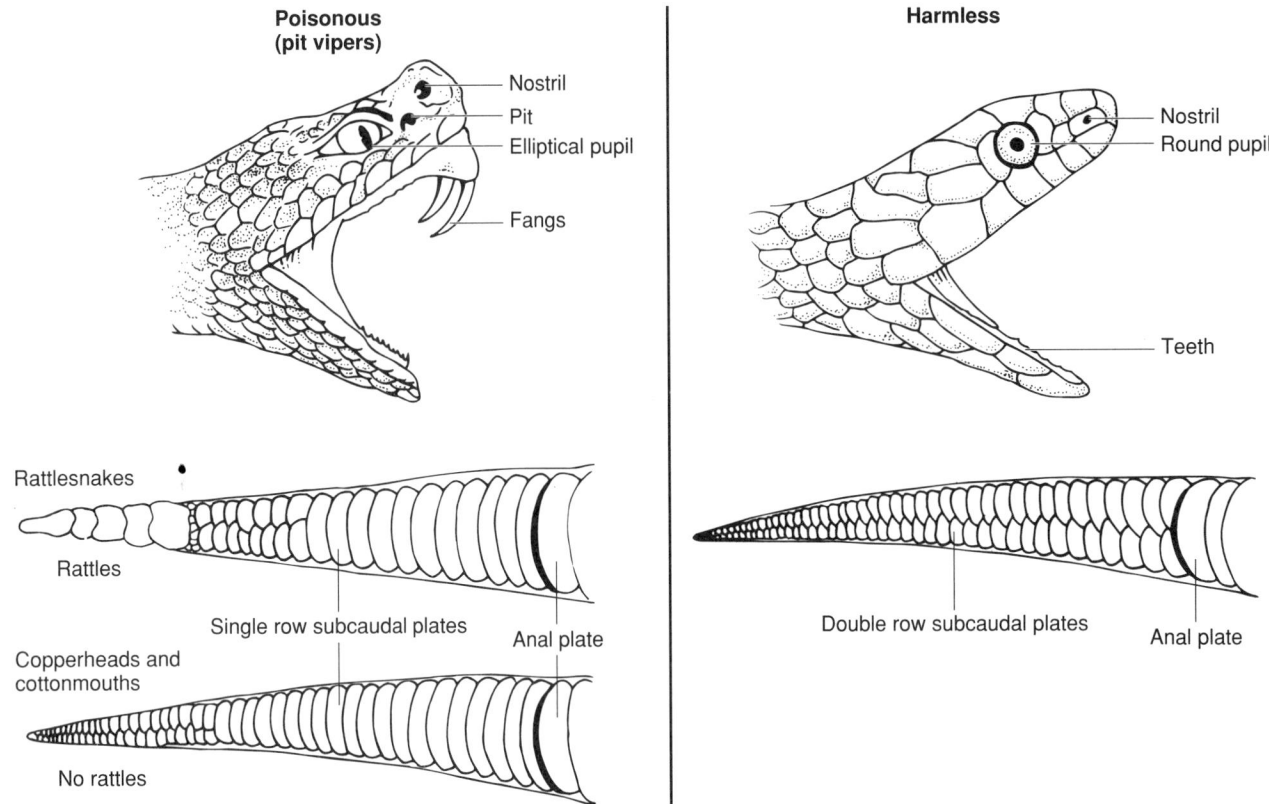

Figure 5-1.
Characteristics that differentiate poisonous pit vipers from nonpoisonous snakes.

bites are painful, and fang marks are the external evidence. The depth of the bite is generally one-third of the distance between fang marks.

Treatment

Treatment of a snakebite includes application of a tourniquet as an emergency measure to prevent lymphatic spread; this is important because almost none of the venom is absorbed through the blood. The distal pulses should be palpable after the tourniquet is applied. Incision and suction for 30 minutes may be beneficial if accomplished within 30 minutes after the snakebite. For severe envenomations, wide excision within 1 hour from the time of the bite can remove most of the venom, obviating the need for antivenin.

Antivenin contains horse serum. There is one **antivenin** for all pit vipers (antivenin *Crotalidae* polyvalent). An antivenin against the venom of the coral snake has been developed, but it is ineffective in treating the bites of coral snakes found in Arizona and New Mexico.

Chapter 6

Hemostasis and Coagulation

Normal hemostasis and coagulation depend on a delicate balance of locally responsive mechanisms operative at the site of vascular injury, the coagulation cascade, and a series of events that terminate clotting and keep it localized. Hemostasis after injury occurs in three phases: (1) reflex vasoconstriction, (2) platelet aggregation and plug formation, and (3) coagulation and clot retraction.

PHASES OF HEMOSTASIS AFTER INJURY

Vasoconstriction

Immediately after injury, the first response designed to control hemorrhage is contraction of the blood vessel wall, which reduces the diameter of the vessel and thus the size of the opening. Vasoconstriction also occurs in response to **thromboxane A$_2$**, a product of arachidonic acid metabolism in platelet membranes. Thromboxane A$_2$ also activates platelets and causes aggregation. The principal mechanism of the anticoagulant action of low-dosage **aspirin** is the inhibition of production of thromboxane A$_2$.

Platelets

Endothelial cell damage exposes blood to collagen and other subendothelial tissue to which platelets are prone to adhere. The mechanism of adherence is complex. Plasma von Willebrand factor (vWF) binds specifically to exposed collagen in the subendothelial tissue. Platelets have a receptor (glycoprotein Ib) for the bound vWF, which serves as a bridge between subendothelial tissue and the platelet. Receptor engagement activates the platelet.

Activation results not only in the flattening of the adherent platelet on the damaged tissue but also in degranulation, which releases many factors. New receptors on the surface are then expressed (IIb and IIIa). These receptors bind fibrinogen, which in turn binds other activated platelets together in an aggregate, thereby plugging the defect. Aggregation of platelets does not occur in the absence of fibrinogen. The surface of the activated platelet is also a major substrate for the intrinsic coagulation cascade. Regulation of the platelet activation process is most likely mediated by normal endothelial cells at the boundary of the platelet plug. These endothelial cells produce prostacyclin and tissue plasminogen activator to limit the spread and size of the platelet plug.

Coagulation Cascade

Within the blood are circulating procoagulants that, when activated by a preceding event in the clotting cascade, promote fibrin formation. Classically, there are two pathways for fibrin formation: intrinsic and extrinsic. Physiologically, it is more likely that the two act in concert.

The **extrinsic pathway** causes large amounts of clot to be formed in seconds and is limited only by the amount of tissue thromboplastin released. The **intrinsic pathway** requires several minutes to form a clot and can be blocked by a number of inhibitors (Fig. 6-1). In clinical practice, the extrinsic pathway is monitored by measuring the **prothrombin time (PT)**, whereas the intrinsic pathway is monitored by measuring the **partial thromboplastin time (PTT)** or **accelerated partial thromboplastin time (aPTT)**.

Figure 6-1.
The coagulation system.

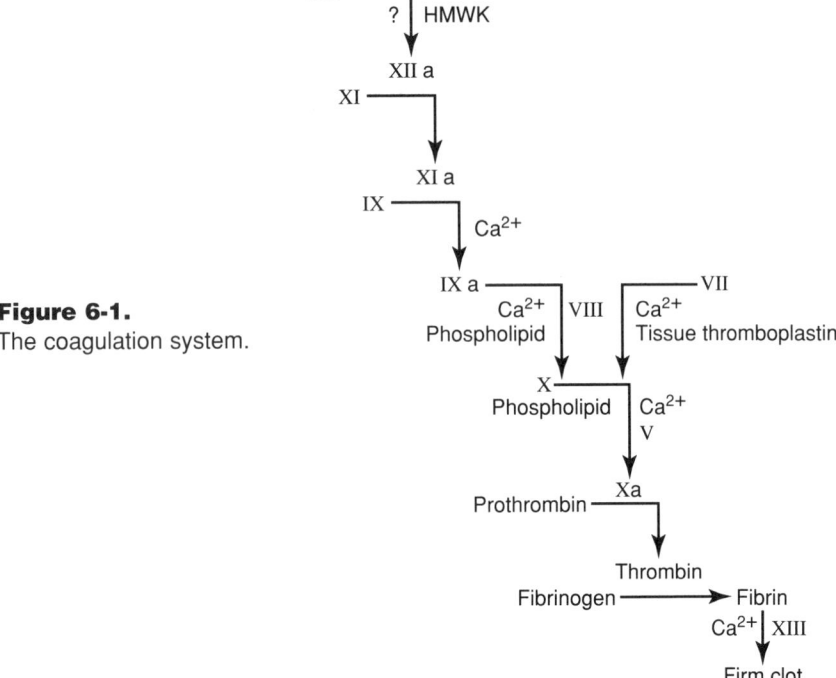

TABLE 6-1.

Clotting Factors

Type	Name	Site of Production	Half-Life (Hours)
I	Fibrinogen	Liver	100
II	Thrombin	Liver (K)	72
III	Tissue factor	Extravascular lipoprotein	
IV	Calcium		
V	Proaccelerin	Liver, endothelium	15
VI	Same as V		
VII	Proconvertin	Liver (K)	4–6
VIII	Antihemophilia factor	Liver, endothelium	8–12
vWF	von Willibrand factor	Endothelium	<10
IX	Christmas factor	Liver (K)	12–24
X	Stuart factor	Liver (K)	50
XI	Plasma Thromboplastin Antecedent	Liver	60
XII	Hageman factor	? Liver	60
XIII	Fibrin-stabilizing factor	? Liver	>100

All procoagulant factors, except vWF, are produced by the liver. **Factors I, VII, IX, and X** share the unique characteristic of having gamma carboxyl glutamic acid in their amino acid sequence and are dependent on **vitamin K** for activation; without vitamin K, they do not undergo gamma carboxylation and are inactive. Table 6-1 summarizes the clotting factors.

Warfarin impairs the formation of vitamin K-dependent factors by reducing the amount of vitamin K available for gamma carboxylation. Clinically, warfarin is followed by observing the PT. Reversal of the effect of warfarin is by administration of vitamin K or by administration of coagulation factors intravenously. **Heparin** is another anticoagulant used clinically. It inhibits coagulation by forming a complex with antithrombin III (AT III). This complex inactivates thrombin and factors VII, IX, X, and XI. Clinically, the effect of heparin is determined by measuring the PTT or aPTT. The **effect of heparin** can be *reversed* by administration of protamine.

DISSEMINATED INTRAVASCULAR COAGULATION

Disseminated intravascular coagulation (DIC) is a syndrome that most commonly occurs in patients who are critically ill with a variety of disorders. In this pathologic condition, activation of the clotting system results in an excess thrombin formation, subsequent fibrin thrombi scattered throughout the body, and a consumption of clotting factors and platelets. DIC may be caused by disease processes that either enzymatically activate procoagulant proteins or cause release of tissue factors that initiate the coagulation process. **Fibrinolysis** occurs subsequent to thrombin formation. Plasmin is formed and fibrin clot is then lysed. DIC can be suspected in the proper clinical setting and with prolonged PT and aPTT, low platelet counts, and decreased fibrinogen levels. The presence of fibrin degradation products, specifically D-dimers in serum, supports the diagnosis.

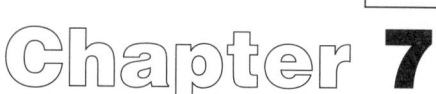

Chapter 7

Blood Replacement Therapy

HEMOSTASIS

Products that augment or replace components of the coagulation cascade are available from blood banks.

FRESH FROZEN PLASMA

Fresh frozen plasma (FFP) is the plasma component of whole blood separated soon after collection and immediately frozen and stored in a frozen state. Most of the coagulation factors approach the concentration in normal plasma when FFP is thawed and infused. The longer the interval between thawing and infusing, the greater the loss of factors V and VIII. None of the factor in FFP is in a greater concentration than normal. Therefore, FFP provides an excellent spectrum of coagulation components, but rather large volumes are required to raise the levels appreciably in recipients. It is the only source of factor V. FFP is a single-donor product with the same risk of transmitting disease as that of whole blood.

CRYOPRECIPITATE

Cryoprecipitate is the next most used aid to coagulation. It is a source of factor VIII and von Willebrand's factor (vWF) and fibrinogen. The major advantage of cryoprecipitate is its small volume and its single-donor status. In practice, pooled units are frequently administered. Platelets are prepared in each blood bank or regional blood center as needed, because platelets cannot be stored for more than a few days. Like cryoprecipitate, platelets are administered as pooled units.

There are various commercially prepared factors available. These include factor VIII concentrate and prothrombin complex concentrate (factors II, VII, IX, and X). Factor VIII is for administration to patients with hemophilia A; factor IX is administered to patients with hemophilia B. The main risk of these products is increased viral transmission of disease (hepatitis; human immunodeficiency virus [HIV] has been eliminated through methods of production).

RED BLOOD CELLS

Eventually, continuing hemorrhage requires transfusion of red blood cells. As red blood cells are lost, there is a diminishing capacity of the blood to carry oxygen. Under proper circumstances, in a person with anemia, half the normal level of hemoglobin can be well tolerated. Patients who are stable should be allowed to replace their own red blood cell mass. Transfusions for anemia are favored when the patient may soon face increased demands or further significant blood loss or when there are preexisting disorders (especially coronary atherosclerosis) that make anemia less well tolerated.

Most red blood cell products are stored in the liquid state in a citrate-based anticoagulant. Citrate binds calcium sufficiently to prevent clotting, is not metabolized during storage, and is a normal intermediary metabolite that is rapidly consumed after transfusion. In addition, the preservation solution contains adenine and glucose, which allows for storage for up to 5 weeks in the liquid state.

RISKS OF TRANSFUSION

Although **ABO incompatibility** is a serious risk, transfusion reactions are usually a result of clerical error. The most frequent serious complication directly attributable to transfusion is the transmission of disease. The most important of these is **hepatitis**. The most serious of the hepatitides is hepatitis C (previously known as non-A, non-B, or NANB). Although hepatitis C is less deadly than hepatitis B, the risk of chronic active hepatitis is higher. Currently, blood is screened for both hepatitis B and hepatitis C, and the risk of acquiring hepatitis has decreased. HIV is also routinely screened, and risk of transmission through blood transfusions is minimal.

Another frequent concern of transfusion is hemostatic breakdown following massive transfusion. It appears that hemostatic breakdown in this setting is primarily a result of shared causes. Rapid and effective restoration of blood volume is probably the most effective way of preventing hemostatic breakdown. There is no evidence that supplementing transfusion of red blood cells with FFP, cryoprecipitate, or platelets prevents this complication.

Other risks of transfusion include transfused cells depleted of 2,3-DPG, causing the oxygen dissociation curve to shift to the left. Although this is a theoretic concern, it has been difficult to demonstrate a harmful effect clinically. Hyperkalemia, citrate toxicity, and metabolic acidosis are also theoretic possibilities. Clinically, however, they rarely manifest. Hypothermia frequently accompanies massive transfusion. In those patients receiving large volumes of banked blood and its components, the products should be warmed before administration.

Chapter 8

Surgical Nutrition

Adequate nutrition is essential for function, growth, and healing. Many surgical patients cannot maintain optimal nutrient intake because of anorexia, depression, gastrointestinal tract obstruction, or dysmotility. Additionally, catabolic stress and metabolic disorders alter nutrient requirements, utilization, or both.

MALNUTRITION

In starving patients, oxygen consumption and metabolic rate are typically reduced, and caloric requirements decline over several weeks to months. The reduced energy requirements are met by mobilization of fat, and a certain level of obligatory **skeletal muscle breakdown** occurs to support **gluconeogenesis**. Hepatic ketogenesis provides an alternative substrate for the central nervous system and other tissues that in a healthy person preferentially oxidize glucose. This metabolic adaptation to chronic starvation allows patients to conserve their most precious metabolic reserve (skeletal and visceral proteins) and expend their generally abundant caloric reserves (fat). In contrast to the whole-body and tissue-specific energy and protein conservation response during unstressed starvation, the injured patient manifests variable but obligatory increases in energy expenditure and nitrogen excretion. The postinjury metabolic environment precludes the efficient oxidation of fat and production of ketones, thereby promoting the continued erosion of protein pools. Unless corrected and treated with organ-specific therapy and nutritional support, critical organs will fail (Fig. 8-1).

PARENTERAL NUTRITION

The majority of surgical patients do not require a special nutritional regimen. Adequate quantities of **parenteral fluids** with ap-

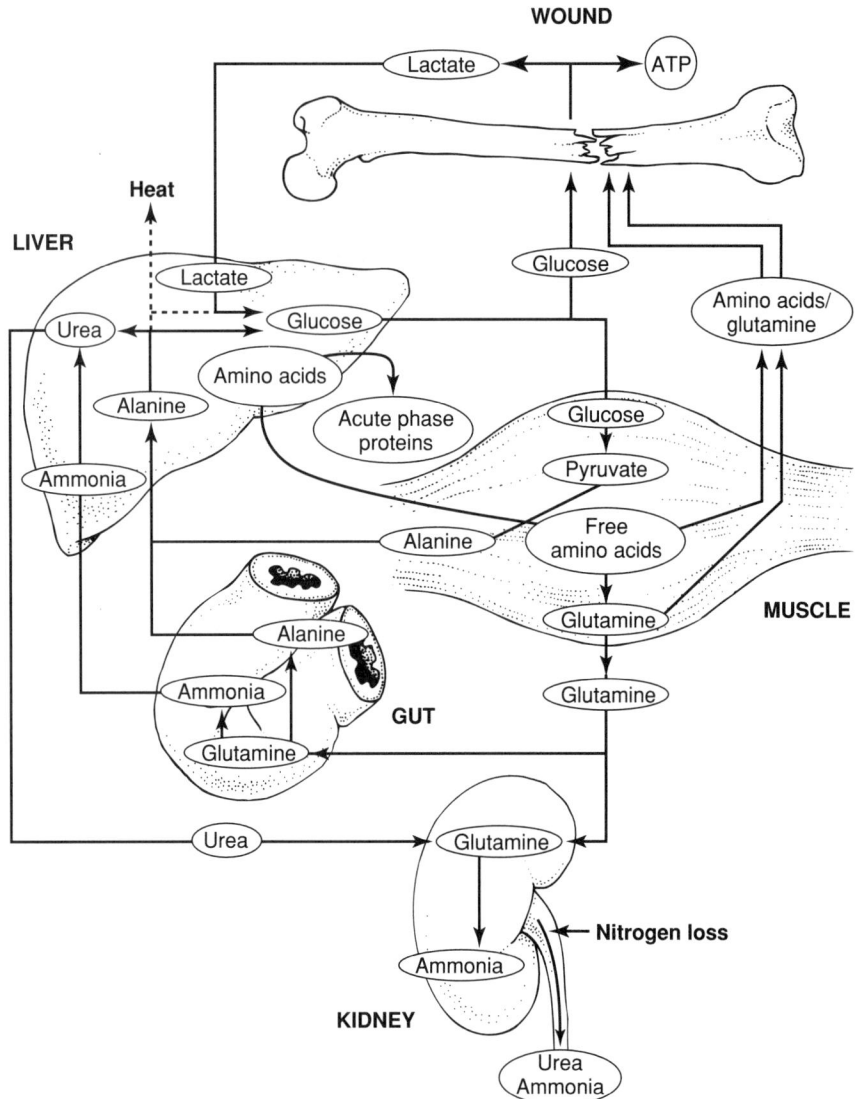

Figure 8-1.
An overall scheme of the metabolic response to stress.

propriate electrolyte composition and a minimum of 100 g of glucose daily to minimize protein catabolism will be all that is necessary in most patients (Table 8-1). In those patients unable to receive adequate oral alimentation but who have a functioning gastrointestinal tract, the preferred method of addressing their nutritional deficiency is by **enteral feeds**. Nasogastric feeding should only be used in alert patients because the risk of aspiration is high in those patients who are unable to protect their airway. A nasoduodenal tube with continuous infusion pumps is preferred in these patients. Percutaneously endoscopically placed gastrostomy (PEG) tubes are a good method of feeding patients with lesions arising above the level of the gastroesophageal junction.

Gastrostomy feedings are contraindicated in mentally obtunded patients. The composition of liquid diets can range from

TABLE 8-1.

Intravenous Requirements (60 to 80 kg Man)

Element	Daily Requirement
H_2O	2000 mL
Na^+	50–90 mEq
K^+	50–100 mEq
Ca^{2+}	1–3 g
Mg^{2+}	20 mEq
Glucose	100 g*

*100 g of glucose minimizes protein catabolism.

elemental preparations to blended foods, based on the patient's requirements.

Parenteral alimentation involves the infusion of a hyperosmolar solution containing carbohydrates, proteins, fats, and other necessary nutrients through an indwelling catheter in the superior vena cava. The indications for parenteral nutrition are broad and encompass a wide range of clinical situations ranging from newborns with catastrophic gastrointestinal anomalies to adults with sepsis syndrome. The clinical setting is very important, and there should always be a specific management goal that administration of parenteral nutrition helps to achieve. It should not be used when gastrointestinal tract feeding is possible. Solutions are commercially available and generally consist of 20% to 25% dextrose, 3% to 5% crystalline amino acids; intravenous lipids are administered at a rate of 2.0 to 2.5 g/kg of body weight. Those patients who do not require a hospital environment for management of their primary disease, yet cannot tolerate adequate enteral or oral feeding, may be candidates for home parenteral nutrition.

Chapter 9

Transplantation

Clinical transplantation replaces diseased organs when they fail and represents one of the greatest successes in surgery and immunobiology in this century. After Alexis Carrel described the technique of vascular anastomosis, the transplantation of primarily vascularized organs became feasible. Rejection occurs in all grafts except those between identical twins, leading to the recognition that individuals possess unique heritable differences in tissue histocompatibility antigens. Within the past 40 years, transplantation of heart, lungs, kidneys, liver, and pancreas have become clinically accepted therapeutic approaches for a wide variety of disease states.

TYPES OF GRAFTS

In general, the greater the genetic difference between graft and recipient, the more vigorous the rejection response. **Allografts** are organ grafts between individuals of the same species; these are rejected with a vigor proportional to the degree of genetic disparity between individuals. Grafts between individuals of different species (**xenografts** or **heterografts**) are rejected even more rapidly. Grafts between identical twins (**isografts**, isogeneic grafts, syngeneic grafts) or from individuals to themselves (**autografts**) survive indefinitely after the vascular supply has been reestablished (Table 9-1).

GRAFT REJECTION

The rejection of an allograft is elicited by foreign histocompatibility antigens on the cell surfaces of the grafted tissue. The strongest of the transplantation antigens is the expression of a single chromosome region called the **major histocompatibility complex**

TABLE 9-1.

Types of Transplant Grafts

Prefix	Meaning
Allo	Transplant between individuals of *same* species
Iso	Transplant between *identical* individuals
Auto	Transplant from an individual to himself or herself
Xeno	Transplant between individuals of *different* species

(**MHC**), which is located on **chromosome 6**. In humans, the gene products of the MHC were first investigated on leukocytes and are called **human leukocyte antigens (HLA)**.

IMMUNOSUPPRESSIVE AGENTS USED IN TRANSPLANTATION

The first agents used for clinical immunosuppression were a combination of corticosteroids plus agents with antiproliferative activity (Fig. 9-1). Most of the agents with antiproliferative activity were adapted for use in cancer therapy. These primarily included antimetabolites (purine analogs such as azathioprine; folic acid antagonists such as methotrexate) and alkylating agents (e.g., cyclophosphamide). Recently, the introduction of new agents (e.g., cyclosporin, OKT3 [a monoclonal antibody], FK506, and ra-

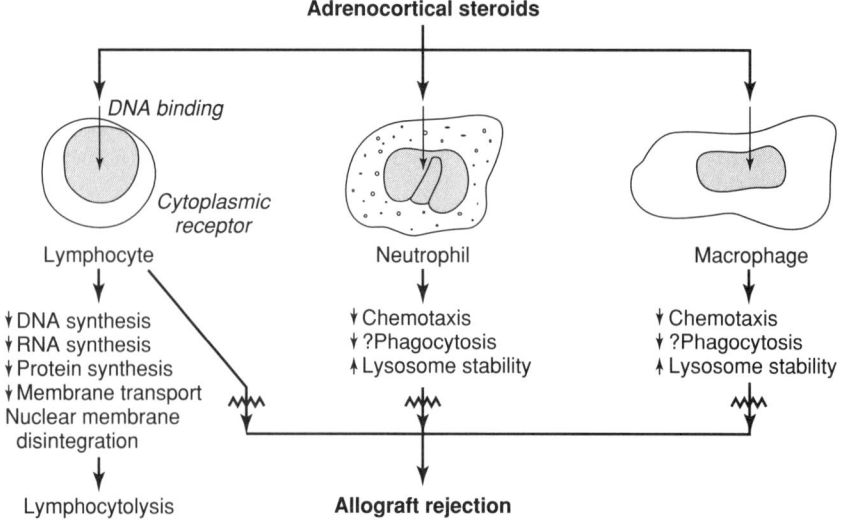

Figure 9-1.
Role of adrenocorticosteroids in clinical allograft immunosuppression.

TABLE 9-2.

Mechanism of Action of Immunosuppressive Agents Used in Transplantation

Agent	Mechanism of Action
Azothioprine	Purine analog; interferes with DNA synthesis
Methotrexate	Folic acid antagonist; inhibits DNA and RNA synthesis
Cyclophosphamide	Alkylating agent; inhibits DNA and RNA synthesis
Cyclosporin	Inhibits T-cell activation and maturation
Antilymphocyte globulin (ALG)	Sera directed against T lymphocytes
Steroids	Produce a decrease in total lymphocytes
OKT3	Monoclonal antibody that binds to T-cell receptor complex (CD3)
FK506	Inhibits T-cell activation and maturation
Rapamycin	Inhibits T-cell activation and maturation

pamycin) that specifically influence T lymphocytes, which are primarily responsible for most graft rejection, has radically changed both the principles of immunosuppression in the organ allograft recipient and the outcome after transplantation. Table 9-2 lists agents currently available. A combination of agents, which each function by a different mechanism, has been found to allow maximal immunosuppression with minimal side effects because a lower dose of each is required.

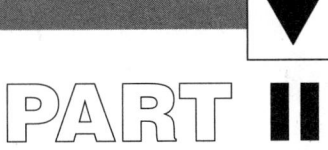

PART II

Specific Surgical Principles

Chapter 10

Head and Neck

Thyroglossal Duct Cysts

The thyroid gland originates from the pharyngeal floor at the **foramen cecum** during the fourth week of gestation. It enlarges, becomes bilobed, and descends ventrally in the midline of the neck in close approximation to the hyoid bone. During its descent, the patent diverticulum is called the thyroglossal duct. The duct normally resorbs by the 10th week of gestation. When all or part of this duct persists, thyroglossal duct cysts or sinuses are formed. Classically, these cysts are midline masses in childhood; 80% occur just **below the hyoid bone**. A maneuver to differentiate them from the Delphian lymph nodes or other central masses is to have the patient protrude the tongue; a thyroglossal duct cyst elevates with tongue movement. Unlike branchial cleft cysts, thyroglossal duct cysts do not have external sinuses. Thyroglossal duct cysts should be removed with a central portion of hyoid bone to prevent recurrence.

Branchial Cleft Anomalies

Branchial cleft cysts, sinuses, and cartilaginous remnants result from the incomplete fusion of the branchial clefts. The branchial clefts, appearing in week 4 of embryonic life and normally involuting fully by week 7, contribute to the formation of various head and neck structures in the developing embryo. When a portion of the cleft persists, epithelial lined cysts or sinuses (with or without cutaneous openings and cartilaginous rests) may manifest. The most common type of branchial cleft anomalies are those of the second cleft, which are present at the middle and lower thirds of the sternocleidomastoid muscle. Excision of these cysts and sinuses is recommended to avoid the complications associated with recurrent infection.

FACIAL FRACTURES

Midfacial fractures usually involve both maxillae and the paired palatine bones. In 1900, Le Fort classified these fractures as follows.

Types of Fractures

Le Fort I fractures (transverse maxillary fracture of Guerin): The fractured segment contains the upper teeth, palate, lower portions of the pterygoid processes, and a portion of the wall of each maxilla.

Le Fort II fractures (pyramidal fractures): In addition to the above, these fractures also contain the nasal bones and the frontal processes of the maxilla. The malar bones are usually not displaced with this fracture. Significant widening of the inner canthi of the eyes and the bridge of the nose usually occurs with this fracture, and there is often destruction of the ethmoid sinus cells.

Le Fort III fractures (craniofacial disjunction): The maxillae, nasal bones, the zygomatic compound are separated as a unit from the cranial attachments (Fig. 10-1). Diagnostic features of these upper jaw fractures include malocclusion, open-bite deformity, and mobility of the upper jaw and hard palate (when the teeth are grasped between the examiner's thumb and index finger).

Stereoscopic roentgenograms in the Waters' position provide excellent visualization of facial fractures. Enhancements in imaging

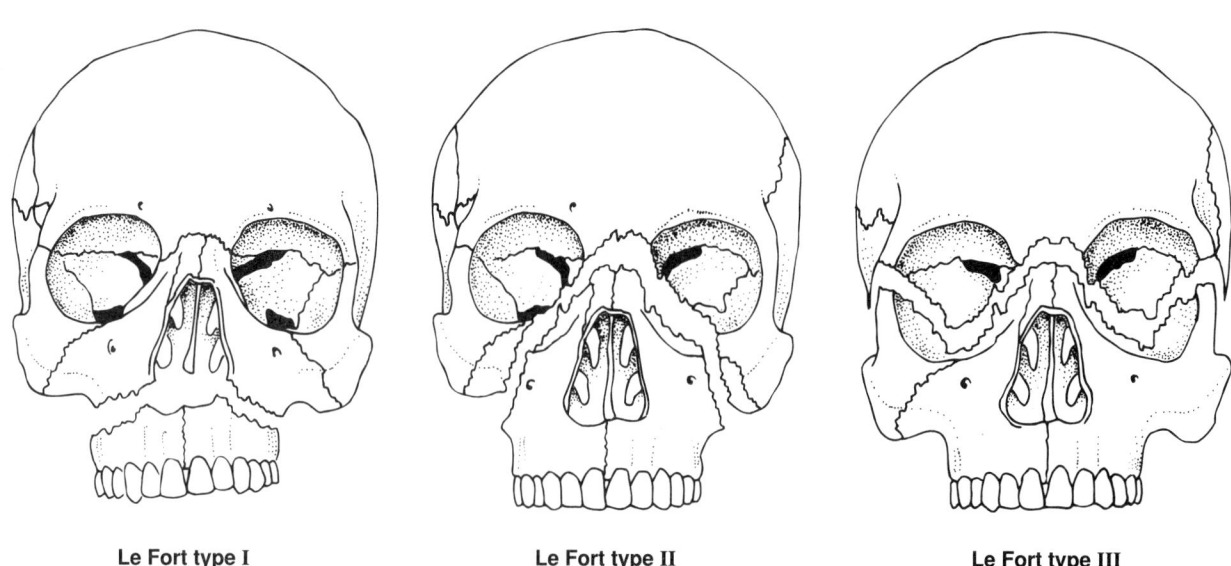

Le Fort type I   Le Fort type II   Le Fort type III

Figure 10-1.
Le Fort types I, II, and III fracture lines as seen in the frontal view.

techniques (computed tomography [CT] scans) have allowed more accurate diagnosis and management of facial fractures. Treatment of these fractures is best accomplished by direct surgical exposure.

HEAD AND NECK CANCER

Tumors

Malignant neoplasms that arise in the head and neck area and upper aerodigestive tract share the general behavior of most solid tumors, which includes local growth, regional spread, and distant metastases. Their effect on disrupting the function of the human organism both before therapy and as a consequence of therapy, however, is more than most other neoplasms. The two main vegetative functions of the human, alimentation and respiration, are often affected by disruptive invasive cancers of the head and neck. Recurrent aspiration pneumonia, malnutrition, upper airway obstruction, and deranged ingestion and speech problems are frequently associated with head and neck cancer. Thus, unlike malignancies of other solid organs, which infrequently cause death from locoregional disease, as many as **60%** of patients with head and neck cancers **die without distant metastases**.

Most malignant tumors that develop in the anatomic area above the clavicles are squamous cell carcinomas, arising from the respiratory tract and stratified squamous epithelium of the upper aerodigestive tract. Collectively, head and neck carcinomas account for 23 new cases per 100,000 males and 8 per 100,000 females in the United States. Incidences and mortality rates in the United States have remained relatively stable over the past 40 years in white men but have increased in nonwhite men and women. **Men** older than 40 years of age with a history of **tobacco and alcohol abuse** comprise **70% to 80% of most patients with head and neck cancer**. Symptoms referable to the tumor itself are usually mild and not commensurate with the size of the tumor. Late-stage presentation is common in these patients.

Diagnosis

Visualization of the entire upper aerodigestive tract is essential for diagnosis. A systematic approach that includes facial and cervical surface anatomy and contour inspection, intraoral examination, and indirect (mirror) laryngoscopy with nasopharyngoscopy is essential for diagnosis and staging. Examination of the neck reveals the presence or absence of metastatic lymph nodes. Tumors with no evidence of primary lesion present as **lymph node metastases in 3% to 4% of malignancies**. A careful physical examination also includes a detailed neurologic examination. Because of the significant incidence of **synchronous primary lesions**, bronchoscopy, esophagoscopy, and direct laryngoscopy are effective in diagnosis. CT and magnetic resonance imaging (MRI) are also helpful in determining the extent of the local or locoregional spread of the tumor.

Therapy

Decisions concerning therapy are based almost completely on the clinical stage of the tumor at the time of presentation. Definitive or curative methods of treatment are oriented toward **total extirpation of local and locoregional disease**. Definitive therapy may consist of excision alone, radiotherapy alone, excision with radiotherapy as a preoperative or postoperative adjuvant, or chemotherapy in conjunction with surgery and radiotherapy. For small tumors (less than 2 cm, T1), surgical removal or radiotherapy provides equivalent local control and improves the survival rate in most cases. As the size of tumor increases (T2 or greater), the likelihood of local control and ultimate cure with radiotherapy alone decreases, so excision or excision with adjuvant radiotherapy is preferable. **Palliative procedures**, which may produce relief of pain, relief of airway obstruction, or improvements in local function and hygiene, also require the complete resection of local disease and may be justified even in the presence of distant disease.

SALIVARY GLANDS

The major salivary glands are the symmetrically paired parotid, submandibular, and sublingual glands, which discharge saliva into the oral cavity via Stensen's ducts, Wharton's ducts, and numerous small orifices in the floor of the mouth, respectively. Numerous other small minor salivary glands are located on the soft and hard palates. The normal volume of **salivary secretion** in men ranges from **1000 to 1500 mL daily**, primarily in the form of serous fluid from the parotid and submandibular glands. Immunoglobulins A, G, and M; albumin; lysozyme; amylase; and other enzymes are secreted. In addition to lubricating properties, saliva has antibacterial and antiviral properties, which protect the soft tissues of the mouth and teeth.

The clinical problem most frequently presented is that of a discrete **mass** in the salivary gland, particularly the **parotid**. A total of 70% to 80% of salivary gland tumors are present in the parotid. Of parotid gland tumors, 80% are benign; of the benign tumors, 80% are **pleomorphic adenomas**. This tumor occurs most frequently during the fifth decade of life, with a slight female predominance.

The second most common benign neoplasm of the salivary glands is the papillary cystadenoma lymphomatosum, or **Warthin's tumor**. Warthin's tumor comprises 4% to 8% of parotid tumors. Facial nerve palsy in parotid tumors is almost never seen, and the presence of such palsy should indicate a malignant tumor. Other signs of malignancy include pain, fixation to surrounding structures, or lymph node involvement. If a lesion is suspected to be malignant, fine-needle aspiration (FNA) should be performed. Surgical treatment of a salivary gland mass is predicated on the assumption that it is malignant.

THYROID

Thyrotoxicosis

Thyrotoxicosis refers to a spectrum of clinical manifestations that are related to an **excess secretion of active thyroid hormone** (Table 10-1). There are three primary types of pathologic processes associated with thyrotoxicosis: Graves' disease (toxic diffuse goiter), toxic multinodular goiter, and single toxic adenoma. The onset of symptoms and signs related to an excess amount of circulating thyroid hormone differs for the three main pathologic processes.

Graves' disease most commonly becomes clinically apparent in young patients, with a male to female ratio of 1:6. Clinically, Graves' disease is characterized by the classic triad of goiter, thyrotoxicosis, and exophthalmos. Excess secretion of T_4 alone does not produce exophthalmos; rather, it is due to the autoimmune aspects of the disease. Thyrotoxicosis of the multinodular goiter usually manifests

TABLE 10-1.

Symptoms and Signs of Hyperthyroidism

Symptoms	Signs
Irritability, emotional lability	Tremor
Sweating, heat intolerance	Warm, moist skin
Palpitations	Tachycardia, atrial fibrillation
Shortness of breath	Heart failure
Increased appetite	Myopathy
Diarrhea	Lid retraction, lid lag
Pruritus	
Menstrual irregularity	

after age 50 years and is more common in women. **Toxic adenoma** occurs in the third to the fifth decades.

Thyrotoxicosis is characterized by a decrease or absence of circulating thyroid stimulating hormone (TSH), as well as elevated T_4 and/or T_3 concentrations in the serum. A high titer of thyroid autoantibodies is also found in many patients with Graves' disease.

Treatment

Definitive treatment may be effected with antithyroid drugs, radioactive iodine, or **surgical excision** of thyroid tissue. In young patients with Graves' disease and in those who are pregnant or lactating, antithyroid drug therapy (**propylthiouracil**) is used initially. **Radioactive iodine** (^{131}I) is usually used in the treatment of older patients. If prolonged drug therapy is required, or if recurrence follows discontinuation of drugs, then thyroidectomy or radioactive iodine is usually indicated. **Subtotal thyroidectomy** may represent the treatment of choice in young adults with severe disease and large goiters, or in patients in whom a rapid response is desirable. The preferable treatment for hyperfunctioning adenomas is surgical excision.

THYROIDITIS

Inflammatory processes of the thyroid may be acute or chronic. Acute thyroiditis is further subdivided into suppurative and nonsuppurative forms. Chronic thyroiditis includes Hashimoto's disease, DeQuervain's thyroiditis, and Riedel's thyroiditis.

Acute Suppurative Thyroiditis

Acute suppurative thyroiditis is the least common form of thyroiditis and usually occurs after upper respiratory tract infections in children and adolescents. The disease is characterized by sudden onset of severe pain in the thyroid and anterior neck, accompanied by dysphagia, fever, and chills. The process is usually unilateral. The most common cause is bacterial invasion by streptococci or staphylococci. Treatment consists of antibiotics and drainage of the abscess, if present.

Hashimoto's Disease

Hashimoto's disease is also known as chronic lymphocytic or autoimmune thyroiditis and is one of the most common **autoimmune** thyroid disorders. It is also the most common cause of **hypothyroidism**. The basic cause of the disease is thought to be a disturbance in immune regulation, in which cytotoxic antibodies combine with complement and killer T cells and attack the thyroid. The incidence is 1 in 1000 patients per year in the United States, and it affects women 15 times as often as men. Patients are usually between the ages 30 to 50 years. Treatment with thyroid hormone suppression is indicated if the gland is symmetric and nonnodular and if the patient is without symptoms. If carcinoma is suspected, surgical intervention is indicated.

De Quervain's Thyroiditis

De Quervain's thyroiditis, or subacute granulomatous thyroiditis, is an uncommon disease that has an incidence approximately one-eighth that of Graves' disease. It is 5 times more common in women, and it is most common in those between the ages of 20 and 40 years. The clinical manifestations include fever, malaise, and unilateral or bilateral thyroid pain. Thyrotoxicosis is present in 50% of cases. The patient's history often includes a recent viral illness. Treatment consists of aspirin or nonsteroidal antiinflammatory drugs (NSAIDs) for pain relief. Steroid drugs can be used if symptoms persist.

Riedel's Thyroiditis

Riedel's thyroiditis is extremely rare and of unknown etiology. It also is known as Riedel's struma or invasive fibrous thyroiditis. The hallmark of this disease is a woody, hard thyroid caused by fibrosis, which usually extends into surrounding neck structures. Compression symptoms occur with progression of the fibrotic process. Surgical intervention may be required for compressive symptoms or to exclude a malignant process.

Solitary Thyroid Nodule

Solitary nodules are clinically present in 4% to 6% of patients in the United States. **Cancer of the thyroid** occurs with an incidence of 50 new cases per 1 million in the United States (approximately 12,000 new cases yearly). By far, most thyroid nodules are benign, with males having fewer benign lesions than females. Previous exposure to radiation and being older than 40 years of age for men and older than 50 years of age for women increases the likelihood of malignancy. Scintillation scanning localizes the site of radioactive iodine (^{123}I) or ^{99m}Tc pertechnetate. Nodules in the thyroid can be hyperfunctional or hypofunctional.

Classes of Thyroid Cancer

The four major classes of thyroid cancer are (1) papillary, (2) follicular, (3) medullary, and (4) anaplastic. In addition, the thyroid may be involved with lymphoma and metastatic carcinoma. In the United States, **papillary** carcinoma comprises two-thirds of all thyroid cancers, **follicular** cancer represents 18%, medullary cancer less than 10%, and anaplastic cancer 10% to 15%.

Most carcinomas present as "cold" nodules. FNA of the nodule should follow discovery of nodules. All patients with malignant cells should undergo surgery. All patients with sheets of follicular cells should also undergo surgical intervention because follicular cancers exhibit the same cellular pattern as follicular adenomas and cannot be differentiated by this technique.

Medullary carcinoma of the thyroid is a C-cell **calcitonin**-producing tumor. It occurs in families as part of the **multiple endocrine neoplasia type II** (MEN-II) syndrome (also known as familial medullary carcinoma syndrome and Sipple's syndrome). The MEN syndromes are summarized in Table 10-2.

PARATHYROID

Embryologically, the parathyroid tissue develops in the third and fourth pharyngeal pouches as early as the sixth week of gestation (Fig. 10-2). The paired inferior glands arise from the third pouch and ultimately descend with the thymus toward the inferior pole of the thyroid. The parathyroid glands consist of predominantly chief cells; the other two types of cells are oxyphilic and clear cells. The parathyroids (chief cells) synthesize and secrete **parathyroid hormone (PTH)**. PTH is essential for calcium homeostasis. PTH primarily affects bone and the kidneys. In bone, it stimulates calcium resorption. In the kidneys, it significantly increases the resorption of calcium and 1-hydroxylation of 25-hydroxyvitamin D_3, which in turn enhances intestinal absorption of calcium and phosphates. Release of PTH by the parathyroid glands is through a negative

TABLE 10-2.

Multiple Endocrine Neoplasia Syndrome

MEN-I (Wermer's syndrome)	MEN-II (Sipple's syndrome)	MEN-III
Pituitary	Medullary carcinoma of the thyroid	Medullary carcinoma of the thyroid
Pancreatic	Pheochromocytoma	Pheochromocytomas
Hyperparathyroidism	Hyperparathyroidism	Rare hyperparathyroidism
		Ganglioneuroma phenotype
		Neuromas of the tongue
		Marfanoid habitus

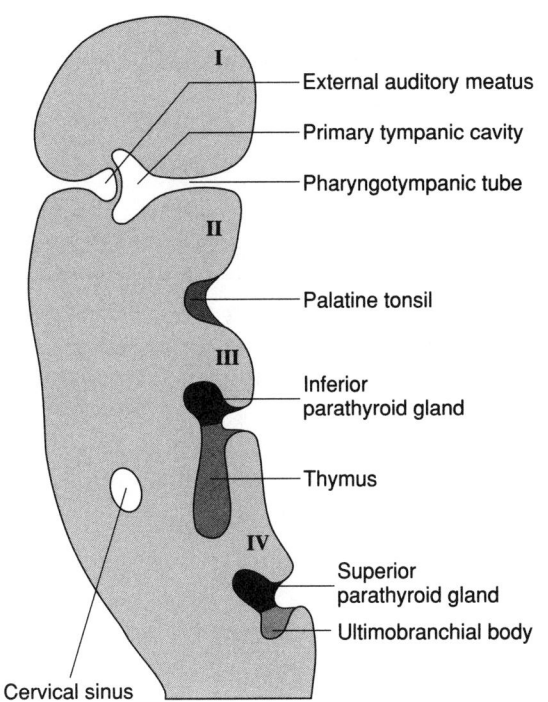

External auditory meatus

Primary tympanic cavity

Pharyngotympanic tube

Palatine tonsil

Inferior
parathyroid gland

Thymus

Superior
parathyroid gland

Ultimobranchial body

Cervical sinus

Figure 10-2.
The development of the
pharyngeal pouches.

feedback system. A fall in serum calcium (or serum magnesium) concentration stimulates secretion of PTH; an elevation of serum calcium reduces both serum PTH and formation of 1,25-hydroxyvitamin D_3.

Surgical intervention is indicated for primary, late secondary, and tertiary hyperparathyroidism (Table 10-3). In **primary hyperparathyroidism**, there is an elevated serum PTH level that does not respond to elevated serum calcium. The most common etiology for primary hyperparathyroidism is a single adenoma or diffuse hyperplasia. The diagnosis is made with elevated circulating levels of intact PTH. In **secondary hyperparathyroidism**, there is also an elevated serum PTH, but this is in response to a lowered blood calcium level, often the result of renal disease or malabsorption syndromes. **Tertiary hyperparathyroidism** is a term that has been used to de-

TABLE 10-3.

Hyperparathyroidism

Type	Serum Calcium	Serum Parathormone
Primary	Increased	Increased
Secondary	Decreased	Increased
Tertiary	Increased	Increased

scribe the condition in which secondary hyperparathyroidism with chief cell hyperplasia appears to have become "autonomous." Normally, there are four glands.

HYPOPARATHYROIDISM

Hypoparathyroidism is seen either as a congenital process or more commonly as a complication of surgical removal of thyroid tissue. It manifests early by paresthesias of the lips and digits, and there may be signs of increased neuromuscular excitability and frank tetany. Treatment consists of a diet high in calcium and vitamin D.

Chapter 11

Breast

The breast is a highly modified sudoriferous gland that develops as ingrowths from ectoderm to form the alveoli and ducts. Located within the superficial fascia of the anterior thoracic wall, the breast is composed of approximately 15 to 20 lobes of glandular tissue. Mammary development and function are initiated by a variety of hormonal stimuli, which include estrogen, progesterone, prolactin, oxytocin, thyroid hormone, cortisol, and growth hormone. During the menstrual cycle, the volume is greatest in the second half of the cycle. The mature breast of the female extends inferiorly from the level of the second or third rib to the inframammary fold at approximately the sixth or seventh rib. Transversely, it extends from the lateral border of the sternum to the anterior or midaxillary line. Greater than 70% of the lymph from the breast passes to the axillary lymph nodes.

Gynecomastia implies the presence of a female-type mammary gland in a male. Most examples of gynecomastia should not be considered disease, because enlargement of the male breast is common. Physiologic gynecomastia occurs most often during three phases of life: (1) neonatal period, (2) adolescence, and (3) senescence. Common to each of these periods is an excess of estrogens in relation to circulating testosterone. Drugs (e.g., digitalis, anabolic steroids, estrogens, marijuana, cimetidine, phenytoin, spironolactone, diazepam, theophylline, verapamil, tricyclic antidepressants, and furosemide), hepatic failure, hyperthyroidism, and hypothyroidism can also induce gynecomastia. Gynecomastia does not predispose the male breast to cancer. For large, progressive gynecomastia refractory to drug discontinuation or therapy for an endocrine defect, the most effective therapy, especially in the young male, is transareolar mastectomy.

BREAST EXAMINATION

The technique of breast examination should include inspection and palpation of the entire breast and draining lymph node sights. Inspection of the breasts should be performed with the clinician standing in front of the patient, with the patient's arms first at the sides and then raised. Symmetry, size, and shape of the breast should be documented as well as any evidence of edema (*peau d'orange*), nipple inversion, skin retraction, or erythema. With the arms extended forward and the patient in a sitting position, a forward lean accentuates skin retraction. Palpation should be conducted with the side to be examined elevated by a pillow, and the breast palpated against the chest wall. Careful palpation of the axillary, cervical, subclavicular, supraclavicular, and parasternal nodes should also be performed. Size, shape, mobility, and consistency of any breast mass or nodal sight should noted.

MAMMOGRAPHY

Mammography should not be used as a substitute for biopsy; rather, this technique is an adjunctive, complementary study that **augments history and physical examination**. Mammography is useful for (1) examination of an indeterminate mass that presents as a solitary lesion suspicious of a neoplasm; (2) examination of an indeterminate mass that cannot be considered a dominant nodule, especially when multiple cysts or other vague masses are present and the indication for biopsy is uncertain; (3) follow-up examination of breast cancer treated by segmental mastectomy and irradiation; (4) follow-up examination of the contralateral breast following total or segmental mastectomy; and (5) evaluation of the large fatty breast in a patient in whom nodules are not palpable (Table 11-1).

TABLE 11-1.

Indications for Mammography

Examination of an intermediate mass that presents as a solitary lesion suspicious of neoplasm

Examination of an intermediate mass that cannot be considered a dominant nodule

Examination of a breast following breast-conservation therapy

Examination of the contralateral breast after mastectomy

Examination of a fatty breast in which masses are not easily palpable

Current guidelines by the American Cancer Society recommend that all women initiate self breast examination at 20 years of age, and that a **baseline** mammographic examination be obtained at 35 years of age after consultation with a physician. In women between the **ages of 40 and 50 years**, mammograms should be obtained under the direction of a physician, and thereafter it is recommended that a mammogram be obtained annually.

BENIGN LESIONS OF THE BREAST

Fibrocystic Breast Disease

Fibrocystic breast disease is an ill-defined entity. Patients often present with diffuse breast pain (mastodynia); pain is accentuated during the second half of the menstrual cycle. Palpation reveals multiple irregularities. **Most lesions are not risk factors** for development of breast cancer. The risk of breast cancer is increased only if there is associated dysplasia. A single dominant cyst (macrocysts, or blue-domed cysts) can be identified by palpation and aspirated. If the aspirate contains blood, the cyst should be excised.

Papilloma

Papilloma presents with a serosanguineous or bloody nipple discharge, usually unilateral. In general, these lesions are quite small and cannot be palpated on examination of the breast. **Intraductal papilloma** is the most common cause of bloody nipple discharge, but it must be distinguished surgically from adenocarcinoma.

Fibroadenoma

The generic term fibroadenoma refers to a benign focal tumor with mixed glandular and mesenchymal elements. Fibroadenomas typically cease growing when they reach 2 to 3 cm in diameter. This lesion has a relationship to estrogen sensitivity and **occurs predominantly in the second and third decades**. On physical examination, the tumor appears to be well encapsulated and is freely movable and not attached to skin or subcutaneous tissue. **Fine-needle aspiration (FNA)** can establish the diagnosis. **Excision to exclude adenocarcinoma** is the preferred treatment, especially in patients older than 35 years of age. The predominant carcinoma that presents concurrently with fibroadenoma is **lobular carcinoma** *in situ*.

CARCINOMA OF THE BREAST

Breast cancer occurs in one of eight women in the United States and is the **second leading cause of death** from cancer in women. Most often the presenting symptom is a **painless lump** that has developed insidiously. In contrast to fibroadenomas, these tumors are not readily movable and can show evidence of infiltration and fixation to the surrounding structures, as manifest by dimpling of the skin, retraction or deviation of the nipple, and elevation of the breast. As the disease progresses, spread occurs in the lymphatics and the axillary nodes become involved early. It is rare, however, for patients with early invasive breast cancer to have clinically detectable distant metastases at the time of initial diagnosis.

Paget's Disease

Paget's disease of the breast presents as a **chronic eczematous eruption of the nipple** and is almost always associated with an **underlying invasive carcinoma**. Symptoms include tenderness, itching, and intermittent hemorrhage. The management of this disease should be the same as any carcinoma of the breast.

Management

The metastatic evaluation should be judicious, consisting of history and physical examination, chest radiograph, measurement of liver function enzymes, and bilateral mammogram. If symptoms suggestive of metastatic disease are present on initial evaluation, further investigations aimed at diagnosing metastatic disease should be obtained. The next goal should be to obtain the diagnosis with the least disturbance of breast tissue. FNA is the simplest, quickest, and most cost-effective approach to establish the breast cancer diagnosis in patients with a **palpable mass**. For **nonpalpable masses** detected by mammogram, stereotactic guidance or ultrasound permits accurate FNA. In most diagnostic centers, the false-negative interpretation is less than 10%; false-positives are rare. A negative or nondiagnostic FNA should be followed by **open biopsy** or biopsy guided by radiologic directed needle placement.

CARCINOMA *IN SITU*

There are two recognized categories of carcinoma *in situ*: **ductal (DCIS) and lobular (LCIS)**. DCIS is part of a biologic continuum that begins with atypical hyperplasia in the ducts, with progression to DCIS and then invasive ductal carcinoma. Patients with surgically excised DCIS are at high risk for developing a subsequent invasive ductal carcinoma in the ipsilateral breast. The standard treatment of DCIS has been **total mastectomy** (often with low axillary nodal dissection). With the detection of smaller tumors (less than 0.5 cm), **breast-conservation therapy** should be considered.

LCIS is not necessarily a component of progressive disease that leads to invasive lobular carcinoma. The presence of LCIS identifies patients who are at high risk for subsequently developing a breast cancer that is more often invasive *ductal* carcinoma rather than lobular. The disease affects all genetically identical breast tissue; therefore, both breasts are at risk for cancer. Options for treatment include **lifelong observation** of both breasts with **mammography and physical examination** or bilateral total mastectomies with consideration of breast reconstruction in selected cases.

GOALS OF TREATMENT

The goals of treatment for breast cancer are (1) cure, (2) local disease control, (3) staging, (4) satisfactory cosmetic result (i.e., minimal disfigurement), and (5) rehabilitation. In many circumstances, variations in surgical treatment do not influence survival.

Three surgical procedures are available for patients with early stage invasive breast cancer: **modified radical mastectomy (MRM)**, **breast-conservation surgery** (lumpectomy, segmental mastectomy) **with irradiation**, and **breast reconstruction** either at the time of mastectomy (immediate) or at some designated time interval (delayed). Numerous randomized prospective trials have demonstrated that survival is not significantly different for patients who have breast-conservation procedures plus irradiation than those who receive MRM for early stage breast cancer.

Contraindications to the breast-conservation approach include multifocal primary tumors, large tumor/breast size ratio, collagen vascular disease, and lack of patient commitment to undergo irradiation and close follow-up. Immediate or delayed breast reconstruction does not interfere with subsequent patient management or detection of regional recurrences. Adjuvant systemic chemotherapy is indicated in patients with node-positive disease and in selected subsets of patients with node-negative histology.

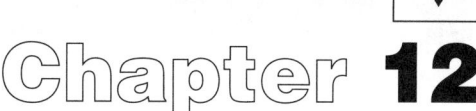

Chapter 12

Thorax and Mediastinum

Trauma

Chest injuries cause one of every four trauma deaths in North America, and many of those patients die after reaching the hospital. Most life-threatening thoracic injuries can be treated with an appropriately placed chest tube or needle. Life-threatening chest injuries include tension pneumothorax, open pneumothorax, massive hemothorax, flail chest, and cardiac tamponade.

Tension Pneumothorax

Tension pneumothorax develops when a "one-way valve" air leak occurs, either from the lung or through the chest wall. The mediastinum and trachea are displaced to the opposite side, decreasing venous return and compressing the opposite lung. A tension pneumothorax is characterized by respiratory distress, tachycardia, hypotension, tracheal deviation, unilateral absence of breath sounds, neck vein distention, and cyanosis as a late manifestation. The most common causes of tension pneumothorax are **mechanical ventilation** with positive end expiratory pressure, **spontaneous pneumothorax** in which **ruptured emphysematous bullae** fail to seal, and **blunt chest trauma** in which parenchymal lung injury has failed to seal. Tension pneumothorax is a clinical diagnosis and should not be made radiologically. Immediate decompression is managed initially by needle decompression (second intercostal space, midclavicular line of the affected hemothorax) and then tube thoracostomy (fifth interspace, anterior axillary line).

Open Pneumothorax

Large defects of the chest wall, which remain open, result in an open pneumothorax or sucking chest wound. Equilibration between intrathoracic pressure and atmospheric pressure is immediate. Effective ventilation is impaired, which leads to hypoxemia. These injuries are managed by promptly closing the defect with a sterile occlusive dressing large enough to overlap the wound's edges. The dressing should be taped on three sides, allowing air to escape as the patient exhales.

Massive Hemothorax

Massive hemothorax results from a rapid accumulation of more than 1500 mL of blood in the chest cavity. This condition is discovered when shock is associated with absent breath sounds and/or dullness to percussion on one side of the chest. Massive hemothorax is most commonly caused by a penetrating wound that disrupts the systemic or hilar vessels. This condition is initially managed with simultaneous restoration of the intravascular volume and decompression of the chest cavity. If more than 1500 mL of blood are present on placement of a 38-Fr chest tube, or if there is ongoing bleeding of more than 200 mL/hour, thoracotomy may be indicated.

Flail Chest

Flail chest occurs when a segment of the chest wall does not have bony continuity with the remainder of the thoracic cage. This condition follows trauma associated with multiple rib fractures. The major difficulty in flail chest stems from the injury of the underlying lung; the defect in the chest wall alone does not cause hypoxemia. Initial therapy includes adequate ventilation, administration of humidified oxygen, and careful fluid resuscitation.

Cardiac Tamponade

This condition most commonly results from penetrating injuries. The human pericardial sac is a fibrous fixed structure, and only a relatively small amount of blood (250 to 300 mL) is required to restrict cardiac activity and interfere with cardiac filling. The classic **Beck's triad** consists of elevated venous pressure, decreased arterial pressure, and muffled heart tones. **Pulsus paradoxus**, a decrease in systolic pressure during inspiration in excess of 10 mm Hg, and **Kussmaul's sign**, a rise in venous pressure with inspiration, may also be present. Pericardiocentesis is the indicated treatment.

MEDIASTINUM

Mediastinal Masses

The mediastinum is the central cavity division of the thorax, bounded on either side by the pleural cavities, inferiorly by the di-

TABLE 12-1.

**Most Common Tumors and Cysts
of the Mediastinum by Location**

Anterior	Middle	Posterior
Thymomas	Cysts	Neurogenic tumors
Benign	Pericardial	Neurofibroma
Malignant	Bronchogenic	Neurilemoma
Lymphomas	Enteric	Neurosarcoma
Hodgkin's disease		Ganglioneuroma
Non-Hodgkin's lymphoma		Ganglioneuroblastoma
Teratodermoids		Neuroblastoma
Benign		Chemodectoma
Malignant		Pheochromocytoma
Germ cell tumors		
Seminoma		
Embryonal carcinoma		
Choriocarcinoma		

aphragm, and merging superiorly with the thoracic inlet. The mediastinum is conveniently divided along anatomic boundaries into subcompartments that contain characteristic lesions. The current classification recognizes three spaces: the **anterior** mediastinum contains the thymus; the **middle** mediastinum contains the heart, pericardium, aorta, trachea and main-stem bronchi, and associated lymph nodes; and the **posterior** mediastinum contains the descending aorta, esophagus, autonomic nerve trunks, and thoracic duct.

Of all mediastinal masses, **primary cysts** (bronchogenic, pericardial, enteric) account for 25% of all masses. Thymic neoplasms (anterior mediastinum) are the most common primary tumors (17%), followed closely by lymphoma (anterior mediastinum) (16%), neurogenic tumors (posterior mediastinum) (14%), and germ cell tumors (anterior mediastinum) (11%). **Lymphoma** is also the most common malignant neoplasm of mediastinal tumors. **Thymoma** is the most common anterior mediastinal mass (Table 12-1). **Surgical intervention** is almost always indicated because it provides definitive diagnosis and frequently provides definitive treatment simultaneously.

Chapter 13

Lng

Cystic Adenomatoid Malformation

Cystic adenomatoid malformation is a cause of respiratory distress in the newborn and can require an emergent operation. Other congenital anomalies, prematurity, and stillbirth are common associations. Surviving neonates present with acute respiratory distress in the first few hours of life. The chest radiograph shows a **multicystic "Swiss cheese" configuration** with overexpansion of the involved region and mediastinal shift toward the normal lung. The pattern seen on chest radiograph can sometimes be confused with congenital diaphragmatic hernia. The prognosis is excellent with successful surgery.

Pulmonary Sequestration

Pulmonary sequestration is a condition in which a portion of the lung, isolated during development from the remainder of the lung, receives its blood supply from an aberrant branch of the aorta instead of from the pulmonary artery. The sequestered lobe is prone to develop **recurrent infections**. If sequestration is suspected, an arteriogram should be performed to confirm the diagnosis and define the aberrant systemic blood supply. A barium esophagogram should also be performed to exclude the possibility of a communication with the esophagus. Operative resection of the sequestration is the treatment of choice.

PULMONARY INFECTIONS

Lung Abscess

A lung abscess is a focus of infection with parenchymal necrosis, usually with cavitation. Distinction between lung abscess and consolidated pneumonia is made as areas of cavitation appear on the chest radiograph and as the peripheral margins of the infection develop sharper definition. Aspiration remains the most common cause of lung abscess. Primary treatment of lung abscesses consists of **antibiotics and drainage**. Based on sensitivities of the infecting organism, antibiotics are administered in high doses intravenously. In the most fortunate cases, spontaneous drainage by expectoration is adequate; spontaneous drainage can be augmented with bronchoscopic aspiration. When antibiotics and internal drainage are ineffective, external drainage or pulmonary resection may be indicated.

Empyema

Empyema is a **suppurative infection** confined to a natural anatomic space by normal epithelial boundaries. In a thoracic cavity, this is the potential space existing between the visceral and parietal pleura. Although empyema is most frequently associated with pneumonia, it can also occur after trauma, pulmonary infarction, or pulmonary resection and can be caused by spread from an intraabdominal source. In the postantibiotic era, empyema has become a less frequent complication of pneumonia and now occurs in less than 1% of cases.

Empyema should be suspected in a patient with a **febrile illness** and **pleural effusion** on chest radiograph. Thoracentesis with Gram's stain and culture of fluid confirms diagnosis and guides selection of antibiotics. Pleural fluid with pH less than 7.20 and glucose less than 40 mg/dL strongly suggests empyema requiring drainage. Successful treatment is based on early diagnosis and adequate drainage. When an **abscess develops**, **open thoracotomy and adequate drainage** usually lead to expansion of the lung and obliteration of the cavity. Decortication and thoracoplasty may be necessary for cure.

BRONCHOGENIC CARCINOMA

Cigarette smoking is the predominant factor in the etiology of lung cancer. Lung cancer now has the highest mortality rate of any cancer in both men and women.

Types of Lung Cancer

Bronchogenic carcinoma is divided into two groups: **small cell lung cancer (SCLC)** and **non-small cell lung cancer (NSCLC)**. Untreated SCLC (**oat cell**) has the most rapidly adverse clinical course of any type of pulmonary tumor, with a median survival time from time of diagnosis of only 2 to 4 months. In NSCLC, there are several histopathologic subtypes: squamous cell carcinoma, adenocarcinoma, large cell carcinoma, and adenosquamous carcinoma. The subclassifications of

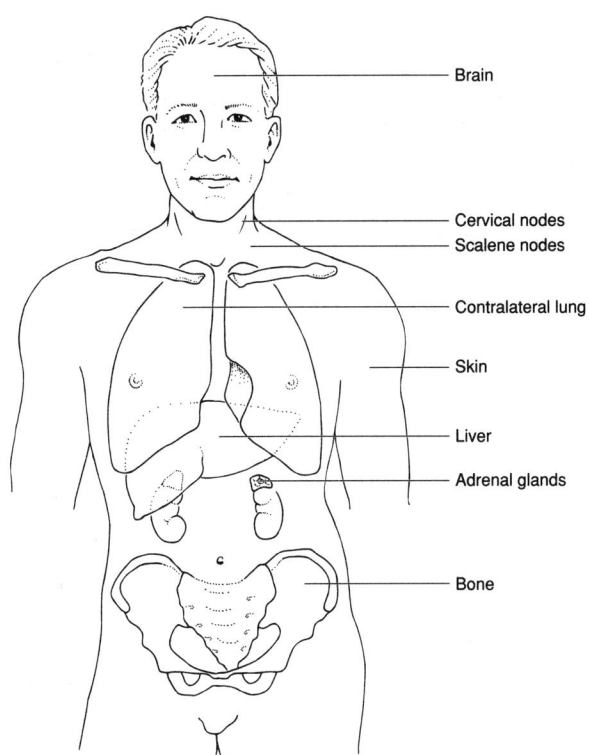

Brain

Cervical nodes
Scalene nodes

Contralateral lung

Skin

Liver

Adrenal glands

Bone

Figure 13-1.
Common sites of
metastases from carci-
noma of the lung.

NSCLC should not be overinterpreted, however, as the therapeutic decision is made largely on the basis of nodal metastases and other aspects of clinical behavior rather than the specific label assigned.

Bronchogenic carcinoma is seen predominantly in men 45 to 65 years of age, with a peak incidence at ages 55 to 60 years. Because intermittent or chronic cough is so common among those who use tobacco, it may be difficult to establish an onset of symptoms. Nevertheless, 75% of patients with bronchogenic carcinoma have **cough** as their principal symptom. **Hemoptysis** is seen in 50% of all patients. Localized **chest pain** is seen if there is invasion into the chest wall. Involvement of the left recurrent laryngeal nerve may result in hoarseness. **Dyspnea** may be due to pleural effusion, invasion of the phrenic nerve, or obstruction of a major bronchus. Weight loss, fatigue, and paraneoplastic syndromes occur in some patients.

Diagnosis and Treatment

Diagnosis of bronchogenic carcinoma is suspected by the presence of a nodule/mass on chest radiograph. The first goal on suspicion of bronchogenic carcinoma is to ascertain potential resectability. At the time of initial presentation, more than 50% of patients are unresectable. It is imperative that **metastatic disease** be evaluated because **surgical resection** is the only likelihood for cure in these patients. A careful history and physical examination may provide clues to metastases. A computed tomography (CT) scan should be done to assess for presence of additional nodules and nodal spread as well as to evaluate the tumor. Bone scan, CT of the head, and nodal biopsy should be performed to confirm metastatic spread (Fig. 13-1). Bronchoscopy should be performed on all patients to evaluate for major bronchial involvement and to assess resectability. Surgical treatment of NSCLC is based on tumor stage. All patients with SCLC should undergo **chemotherapy**, regardless of tumor stage.

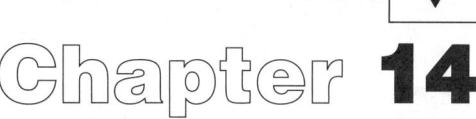

Chapter 14

Heart and Great Vessels

Because rheumatic fever is now rarely seen, congenital heart disease is the **most common form of heart disease seen in children**. In several studies, the frequency has been found to be 3 or 4 cases of congenital heart disease occurring in every 1000 births. Congenital heart disease can be classified by the type of anatomic abnormality present, which in turn produces a distinct physiologic defect. Four major groups exist: (1) left-sided obstructive lesions, (2) left-to-right shunts (acyanotic group), (3) right-to-left shunts (cyanotic group), and (4) complex malformations (Table 14-1).

LEFT-SIDED OBSTRUCTIONS

The most common **left-sided** obstructive lesions are **aortic valvular stenosis and coarctation of the aorta.** These impede emptying of the left ventricular chamber, causing **systolic overloading** and corresponding concentric hypertrophy of the ventricle. With severe levels of neonatal obstruction, heart failure is life threatening and emergency operation is required.

LEFT-TO-RIGHT SHUNTS

Atrial septal defects (ASD), ventricular septal defects (VSD), and patent ductus arteriosus (PDA) are examples of **left-to-right shunts.** As pressures in the left atrium and left ventricle are normally greater than in the right atrium and right ventricle, a defect in the atrial or ventricular septum causes a shunt of oxygenated blood from the left side of the heart to the right side of the heart. This causes pulmonary congestion from an increase in pulmonary

```
┌──────────────┐
│ TABLE 14-1.  │
├──────────────┴─────────────────────────────────┐
│ Classification of Congenital Heart Disease      │
└────────────────────────────────────────────────┘
```

Left-sided obstruction
    Aortic stenosis
    Coarctation of the aorta
Left-to-right shunts (acyanotic group)
    Atrial septal defects
    Ventricular septal defects
    Patent ductus arteriosus
Right-to-left shunts (cyanotic group)
    Tetralogy of Fallot
    Transposition of the great vessels
    Tricuspid atresia
    Truncus arteriosus
    Pulmonary stenosis—pulmonary atresia with intact ventricular septum
Complex malformations

blood flow and often a corresponding decrease in systemic blood flow without cyanosis. With increased pulmonary blood flow, pulmonary vascular resistance may increase.

Patent Ductus Arteriosus

Patent ductus arteriosus (PDA) is a persistence of the embryologic shunt from the aorta to the pulmonary artery and is associated with a classic machinery murmur heard along the left sternal border. The treatment of choice is ligation and division of the PDA.

Atrial Septal Defects

Atrial septal defects (ASD) must be **differentiated from patent foramen ovale (PFO),** which is a normal defect in up to 25% of adult hearts. Because of its slit-like opening, the PFO permits shunting only from right to left. ASD are divided into **ostium secundum** and **ostium primum defects**. Ostium secundum defects are more frequent and more readily repaired. (Ostium primum is an older term; the generic term used is either endocardial cushion defect or atrioventricular canal.) **Mitral and tricuspid insufficiency** accompany ostium primum defects. Ostium primum defects are uncommon and present later in life. They are especially common in patients with trisomy 21 (Down's syndrome). Repair is indicated when the shunt is large and the volume of flow in the pulmonary circuit is 0.5 to 2 times greater than the systemic circuit.

Ventricular Septal Defects

Ventricular septal defects (VSD) are the most common congenital malformation of the heart, comprising 20% to 30% of all cases. Small defects should simply be observed because 60% to 70% close before the age of 3 years. The risk of endocarditis is small. The treatment of large defects depends on the presence of cardiac failure and increasing pulmonary vascular resistance. With the safety of operation and the ominous uncertainty of an increase in pulmonary vascular resistance, it is becoming clear that most children with large VSD should undergo operative repair within the first year of life.

RIGHT-TO-LEFT SHUNTS

Right-to-left shunts of venous blood directly into the systemic circulation, producing arterial hypoxemia and cyanosis, result from the combination of intracardiac septal defect with obstruction to normal blood flow into the pulmonary artery. The classic example of this is tetralogy of Fallot, a combination of pulmonary stenosis and VSD. Other cyanotic disorders include pulmonary stenosis-pulmonary atresia with intact ventricular septum, tricuspid atresia, truncus arteriosus, and transposition of the great vessels. Cyanosis is the most prominent feature of right-to-left shunts. It is estimated that 5 g of reduced hemoglobin is required to produce cyanosis. **Peripheral cyanosis** results from a decrease in cardiac output and sluggish regional flow; **central cyanosis** results from a defect in oxygenation of blood in the lungs or an intracardiac shunt.

Tetralogy of Fallot

Tetralogy of Fallot (TOF) is the **most common cyanotic malformation**. The four features of TOF are obstruction of the outflow tract of the right ventricle, a VSD, dextroposition of the aorta, and hypertrophy of the right ventricle. Anomalous origin of the left anterior descending artery is found in 5% of patients. Currently, total correction seems to be a preferable procedure if feasible. A shunt operation is sometimes indicated. The safest and most effective shunt is either the standard Blalock-Taussig subclavian pulmonary anastomosis or a modified Blalock-Taussig subclavian pulmonary PTFE (polytetrafluoroethylene) interposition graft.

ACQUIRED HEART DISEASE

Coronary Artery Disease

Atherosclerosis (AS) is a multifactorial disease that causes the formation of obstructive lesions in the aorta, peripheral vessels, and coronary arteries. AS is the leading cause of death in the Western world, and acute myocardial infarction results in 25% of deaths in the United States each year. **Angina** is the **principal manifestation** of atherosclerotic coronary artery disease. Other frequent symptoms associated with cardiac disease include (1) symptoms of congestive heart failure, (2) arrhythmias, (3) syncope, and (4) fatigue.

Management

Cardiac catheterization remains the gold standard for diagnosis of coronary artery disease. Frequently, the functional status of the heart is evaluated with radionuclide imaging or echocardiography in addition to cardiac catheterization. Current indications for **coronary artery bypass grafting (CABG)** include (1) patients with mild angina, but left main coronary artery disease, and patients with triple vessel disease and depressed myocardial function; (2) patients with moderate to severe angina not responding to medical management; (3) patients with unstable angina; and (4) patients with acute infarction demonstrating evidence of subendocardial infarction or hemodynamic instability and postinfarct patients with left main artery disease or triple vessel disease.

Chapter 15

Esophagus

The esophagus is a muscular tube beginning at the pharynx and ending at the cardia of the stomach. There are three normal areas of esophageal narrowing. The uppermost narrowing is located at the entrance into the esophagus and is caused by the cricopharyngeal muscle; it is the narrowest point of the esophagus. The middle narrowing is due to an indentation of the anterior and left lateral esophageal wall, caused by the crossing of the left mainstem bronchus and aortic arch. The lowermost portion is at the diaphragmatic hiatus and is caused by the gastroesophageal sphincter mechanism (Fig. 15-1).

GASTROESOPHAGEAL REFLUX DISEASE

Gastroesophageal reflux disease (GERD) is a common disorder that comprises 75% of clinical esophageal pathology. Despite its common prevalence, it can be difficult to diagnose. In the past, it was inferred by the presence of a hiatal hernia, later by endoscopic esophagitis, and more recently by a hypotensive lower esophageal sphincter pressure. GERD can be assessed by determining the basic pathophysiologic abnormality; more specifically, **measure the esophageal pH** with a miniature pH probe and data recorder to calculate the number of hours the pH was less than 4 over a 24-hour period.

GERD is treated initially with **antacids** and **lifestyle modifications** such as weight loss, avoidance of alcohol and coffee, avoidance of tight clothing, elevation of the head of the bed, and avoidance of a meal shortly before retiring. The second phase of medical management is **acid suppression**. H_2-blockers or hydrogen potassium proton pump blockade is administered with a course of medication for 6 months. Unfortunately, 80% of patients have recurrence of symptoms.

Surgical therapy to correct the lower esophageal sphincter is indicated when: (1) there is increased esophageal exposure to gastric juice on 24-hour pH monitoring; (2) the lower esophageal

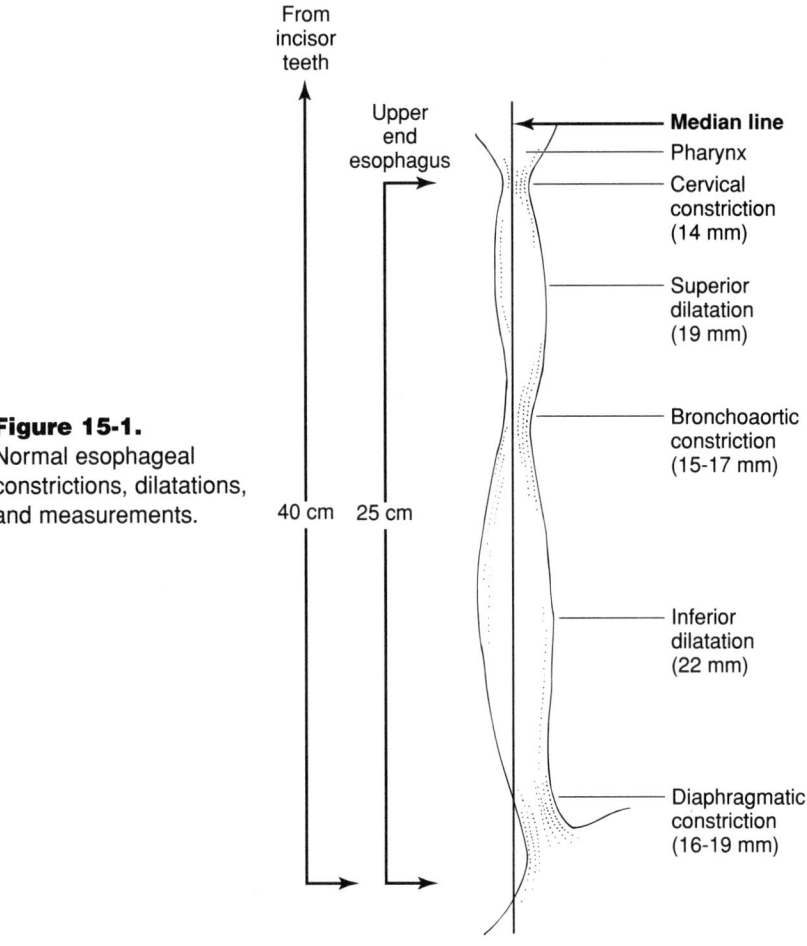

Figure 15-1.
Normal esophageal
constrictions, dilatations,
and measurements.

sphincter is documented to be mechanically defective by manometry studies; and (3) there is adequate esophageal contractility. Sequelae of reflux disease such as anemia, aspiration, and reactive airway disease are also compelling reasons to proceed with antireflux surgery.

Barrett's esophagus is a premalignant condition where the tubular esophagus is lined with columnar epithelium rather than squamous epithelium. This is an acquired abnormality seen in 7% to 10% of patients with GERD.

ESOPHAGEAL CARCINOMA

Esophageal carcinoma is most frequently diagnosed in men between the ages of 50 and 60 years. **Squamous cell** carcinoma accounts for the majority of esophageal carcinomas. Tumors of the lower esophagus and cardia are usually **adenocarcinomas.** The most important etiologic factor in the development of primary adenocarcinoma of the esophagus is **columnar metaplasia** or **Barrett's esophagus**.

Esophageal cancer is a disease affecting patients of advancing age, with dysphagia and weight loss being by far the most common symptoms at the time of diagnosis. In fact, the most common cause of dysphagia in middle age and older is cancer of the esophagus. All patients should be evaluated with a barium swallow or esophagoscopy with biopsy. Patients with tumors of the middle third should also undergo bronchoscopy to evaluate for tracheal involvement. Computed tomography (CT) of the chest is of little value in staging small tumors. The selection of curative versus palliative operation for cancer of the esophagus is based on tumor location, patient age, physiologic fitness, extent of disease, and intraoperative staging.

Chapter 16

Abdomen

ABDOMINAL TRAUMA

The abdominal cavity has three distinct anatomic compartments: the peritoneal cavity, the retroperitoneal space, and the pelvis. The peritoneal cavity can be further subdivided into the upper abdomen, that portion covered by the bony thorax, and the lower abdomen. The upper abdomen includes the diaphragm, liver, spleen, stomach, and transverse colon, whereas the small bowel and remaining portion of the intraabdominal colon are included in the lower abdomen. The retroperitoneal space contains the aorta, vena cava, pancreas, kidneys, ureters, and portion of the duodenum and colon. Injuries to the retroperitoneum are difficult to diagnose because this area is remote from physical examination and is not assessed by **diagnostic peritoneal lavage (DPL)**. The pelvis contains the rectum, bladder, iliac vessels, and in women the internal genitalia. Early diagnosis in these structures is similarly compromised because of anatomic location. In assessing abdominal trauma, the primary factor is not the accurate diagnosis of a specific type of injury but rather the determination that an abdominal injury exists.

The abdominal examination should be conducted in a meticulous, systematic manner in the standard sequence: inspection, auscultation, percussion, and palpation. Any evidence of peritoneal irritation, localization of pain, or blood in the rectum or urethral meatus should be noted. A **positive physical examination** is the most reliable clinical sign of significant abdominal trauma. Further assessment of abdominal injury is by either a **computed tomography (CT) scan** or **DPL**. The only absolute contraindication to these is the pressing need for exploratory laparotomy celiotomy. CT scan and DPL are compared in Table 16-1.

Blunt Abdominal Trauma

Injury patterns from blunt abdominal trauma are different from those of penetrating wounds. The liver, spleen, and kidneys are the organs predominantly involved following blunt trauma, although the relative incidence of hollow visceral perforation and lumbar

	Diagnostic Peritoneal Lavage	Computed Tomography Scan
Time	Faster	
Transport		Required
Sensitive	Greater	
Specific		Greater
Safe	All patients	Stable patients

spinal injuries increases with incorrect seat belt use (lap-belt syndrome). The appearance of **transverse linear ecchymosis** on the abdominal wall (seat-belt sign) or the presence of anterior lumbar compression fracture on radiograph should alert the physician to the possibility of intestinal injury.

Penetrating Injuries

Penetrating injuries may involve indirect effects such as blast and cavitation, as well as the injury incurred as a result of the anatomic course of the missile or weapon inflicting the injury. As expected, the liver, small bowel, colon, and stomach are commonly involved. Stab wounds traverse adjacent structures, whereas gunshot wounds may have circuitous trajectory injuring multiple noncontiguous organs.

Pelvic Fractures

Pelvic fractures often result in significant morbidity and mortality; the most severe pelvic injuries result from automobile accidents involving pedestrians and motorcycles or high-fall incidents. Major hemorrhage from pelvic fractures poses an extremely difficult problem in management. Rectal and genitourinary injuries must be suspected and excluded in all patients with pelvic fractures. The bleeding from pelvic fractures is most effectively controlled by stabilizing the pelvis and allowing the closed retroperitoneal space to tamponade. External pelvic fixation is the currently favored method of rapidly stabilizing a mechanically unstable pelvic ring.

Chapter **17**

Stomach and Duodenum

PEPTIC ULCER DISEASE

Etiology

The etiology of benign gastric ulcer is not completely understood. Prepyloric ulcers have the same secretory patterns as duodenal ulcers—with elevated fasting levels of acid output. In benign gastric ulcers, however, the basal levels of acid secretion are low. In all gastric ulcers, a biopsy is indicated if the ulcer has not responded to therapy. Acute gastritis occurs as a complication of stress, sepsis, burn, or multisystem trauma and represents end-organ failure as part of the multisystem organ failure syndrome.

Duodenal Ulcers

Duodenal ulcer (DU) is generally associated with acid hypersecretion. Chronic DU disease presents in a number of ways. It usually has onset in early or mid-adult years and occurs more frequently in males than in females, with almost no risk of malignancy. Common symptoms include **pain and bleeding**. With recurring exacerbations of ulcers, changes that produce organic complications such as obstruction and perforation may occur. Intractable pain may be an indication for surgery because these patients have been shown to comply poorly with drug treatment.

THERAPY FOR PEPTIC ULCER DISEASE

The need for surgical therapy for peptic ulcer disease has diminished greatly over the past 20 years because of the advent of **H₂-receptor blockers** and, more recently, **hydrogen potassium proton pump** inhibitors. **Surgical therapy** for chronic peptic ulcer has two purposes: (1) to salvage patients from life-threatening complications of perforation, massive hemorrhage, and gastric outlet obstruction, and (2) to provide cure for the disease in the form of protection from recurrence. Therefore, the indications for surgery include perforation, massive bleeding, obstruction, and occasionally intractable pain. In addition, for nonhealing gastric ulcers, suspicion of malignancy is also an indication for operation. Prepyloric ulcers and combined gastric and DU disease are best treated with an acid-reducing procedure such as **truncal vagotomy** and **antrectomy** to include resection of the gastric ulcer. When pyloric obstruction is present, pyloroplasty or gastrojejunostomy is indicated.

Acute gastric ulcer disease usually manifests by **massive hemorrhage**, and treatment is directed toward intravascular resuscitation, control of hemorrhage, and healing of the ulcerative process. In more than 80% of patients, bleeding stops with **gastric lavage** with solutions at room temperature. The stomach must be completely evacuated of blood contents to reduce fibrinolysis at the bleeding sites. In addition, the stomach is stimulated to secrete gastrin if the antrum is distended by clots. The next step is to provide **intragastric neutralization** with H_2 blockers or instillation of antacids into the stomach; the gastric pH should be more than 5. If bleeding persists or recurs, **transendoscopic bipolar electrocautery** of the bleeding ulcer should be attempted. Continued bleeding beyond this point is an indication for **surgery**. At the time of surgery, bleeding ulcers are oversewn and a highly selective vagotomy or truncal vagotomy and pyloroplasty is performed. Some surgeons prefer partial gastrectomy and vagotomy.

Because DU are believed to be the result of gastric hyperacidity, **surgery** is aimed at **decreasing gastric acid production**. These surgical procedures include truncal vagotomy, highly selective vagotomy (parietal cell vagotomy with sparing of the nerves of Latarget), or removal of the gastric antrum (removing the portion of the stomach where gastrin is produced). In truncal vagotomy, some form of drainage of the stomach must be provided because the vagus nerve not only influences gastric acid secretion, but also serves as the motor nerve for the stomach. The surgical procedure with the lowest risk of recurrence of DU is the truncal vagotomy and antrectomy (Fig. 17-1).

In the treatment of **duodenal perforation**, early surgery with closure and oversewing the perforation with an omental patch is indicated. Those who have surgery soon after perforation have a favorable prognosis, whereas those who have had continuing leakage over 12 hours or more have generalized peritonitis and a less favorable prognosis.

Surgery that ablates the pyloric mechanism (vagotomy) may lead to **dumping syndrome**. This syndrome is characterized by feeling faint, sweating, palpitations, and nausea shortly after the ingestion of food. The cause appears to be related to the rapid passage of hyperosmolar liquids into the small intestine. The symptoms result from distention of the intestine and reduction of plasma volume. Hypoglycemia is seen in some patients (late dumping syn-

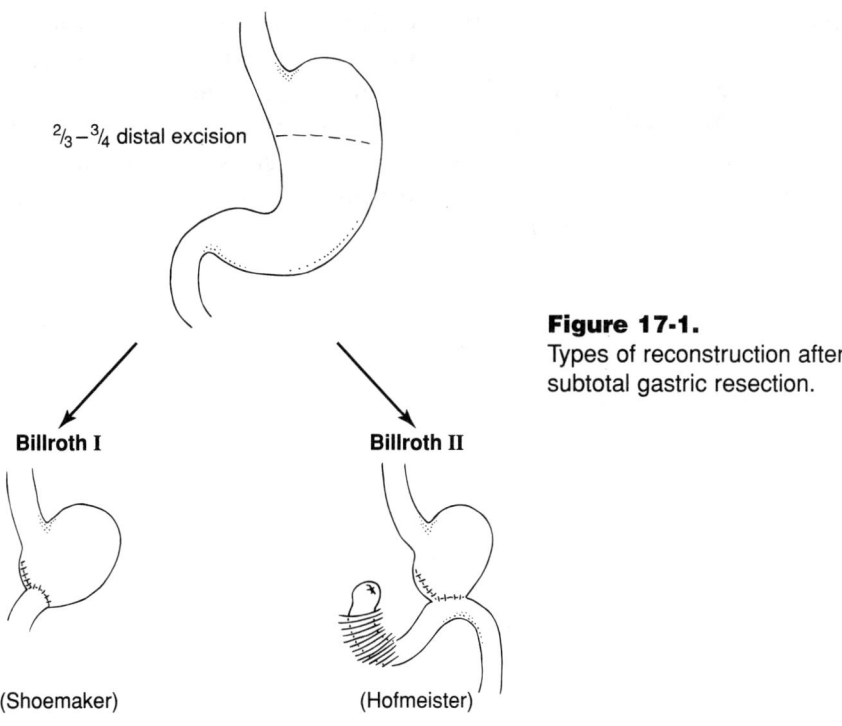

$^2/_3 - ^3/_4$ distal excision

Billroth I

(Shoemaker)

Billroth II

(Hofmeister)

Figure 17-1.
Types of reconstruction after
subtotal gastric resection.

drome). Treatment is directed at reducing the hyperosmolarity of
the material leaving the stomach: fat is increased, carbohydrates are
decreased, and liquids are given between meals.

GASTRIC CARCINOMA

Carcinoma of the stomach has decreased in frequency in the United
States for reasons that are unclear. It occurs twice as often in males
as females. It usually appears at approximately age 45 years and
older, and is characterized by rather indefinite digestive symptoms
such as indigestion, malaise, and lack of appetite. As the disease
progresses symptoms become more marked, with obstruction
(when the tumor is large enough to obstruct the pylorus), bleeding,
and anemia. Many patients with gastric cancer have **pain similar to
that of peptic ulcer disease**. A **carcinomatous ulcer** may appear as
peptic ulcers on barium swallow or gastroscopy. A four-quadrant
biopsy of the ulcer should be obtained.

Treatment

Surgical resection is the only known method of cure for carcinoma
of the stomach. The prognosis is usually poor because by the time

patients are referred for surgery, complete removal of the stomach is not possible because of tumor spread. The extent of stomach removed depends on the operative findings. Although radical gastrectomy has been advocated, there is no convincing evidence that such a procedure produces more positive results, and the morbidity rate associated with total gastrectomy is much greater than that of subtotal resection of the stomach.

Chapter ▼ 18

Gallbladder and Bile Ducts

CHOLELITHIASIS

Calculous cholelithiasis is a chronic disease frequently subject to acute exacerbations known as **biliary colic**. The disease usually occurs during middle life. It is more common in females and often follows pregnancy. **Gallstone formation** is thought to result from abnormalities in the composition of bile. Most important is the maintenance of a normal ratio among bile salts, phospholipids, and cholesterol. An increase in cholesterol or a reduction in the bile salt pool results in "lithogenic bile." The bile salt pool is reduced by resection or bypass of the distal ileum. Asymptomatic cholelithiasis is not an indication for cholecystectomy.

CHOLECYSTITIS

Acute Cholecystitis

If a stone obstructs the cystic duct, an attack of acute cholecystitis may follow. In general, these attacks occur at night and are more likely to follow a dietary indiscretion such as overeating. There is **severe pain**, which presents in the **epigastrium or right upper quadrant**; frequently, it radiates to the back, scapular region, or right shoulder. Nausea and vomiting are common. During the attack, tenderness with guarding is present in the region of the gallbladder. These attacks usually subside after a few hours with the aid of analgesics and antibiotics.

Acute cholecystitis results from acute inflammation of the gallbladder, which usually originates in **bacteria**. The most common pathogens isolated from the bile in acute cholecystitis are

Escherichia coli, Klebsiella, and *Enterococcus.* When identified early, the most appropriate therapy for acute cholecystitis is **cholecystectomy**. The following conditions must be considered in the differential diagnosis of acute cholecystitis: (1) acute appendicitis, (2) perforated peptic ulcer disease, (3) acute pancreatitis, (4) renal colic or pyelonephritis, (5) pneumonia, or (6) myocardial infarction.

Chronic Cholecystitis

The most common presentation for patients with symptomatic gallstones is postprandial right upper quadrant pain. This usually is precipitated by a fatty or protein-rich meal, occurs 30 to 60 minutes after eating, and lasts for several hours and then resolves. This group of symptoms is referred to as biliary colic. It should be noted, however, that in contrast to other forms of colicky pain, which are characteristically intermittent and spasmodic, the **pain** of biliary colic usually is **constant**. It is a self-limiting process and usually resolves within a few hours of onset. Ultrasound documentation of gallstones, with a history consistent with biliary colic, establishes the diagnosis, and cholecystectomy should be performed. Currently, **laparoscopic cholecystectomy** is the preferred surgical method.

BILE DUCT DISORDER

Choledocholithiasis

Gallstones in the common bile duct, which obstruct bile flow, manifest clinically as **jaundice**. Additionally, many patients have associated right upper quadrant pain, fever, and ascending cholangitis (**Charcot's triad**). Laboratory studies show an elevated leukocyte count and elevated liver enzymes and serum bilirubin; this is in contrast to acute cholecystitis, in which liver enzymes and bilirubin are normal.

Initial management includes intravenous fluid resuscitation and antibiotics. For the severely ill patient, endoscopic retrograde cholangiogram or percutaneous biliary stents should be undertaken to decompress the biliary tree and drain the infection. In all cases, **cholecystectomy** eventually is necessary to eliminate the possibility for recurrence. In any patient undergoing cholecystectomy, elevated preoperative liver function studies and/or ultrasound documentation of a common bile duct of greater than 7 mm in diameter should prompt an intraoperative cholangiogram (IOC).

TABLE 18-1.

Diseases of the Gallbladder

Disease	Meaning
Cholelithiasis	Presence of stones in the gallbladder
	Does not imply disease
Cholecystitis	
Acute	Acute inflammation of the gallbladder: (+) Murphy's sign
	Gallstones usually seen on ultrasound
	Usually associated with infection
	Confirmed by an IDA (^{99}Tc-labeled immunodiacetic acid): nonvisualization of the gallbladder
	Acalculous—seen in critically ill patients
Chronic	Also called *biliary colic*
	Characterized by intermittent, recurrent attacks of right upper quadrant or epigastric pain that follows meals
	No fever or acute signs of inflammation are present
	Hydrops: chronic cystic duct obstruction gallbladder distends with mucus *(white bile)*
Choledocho-lithiasis	Stones in the common bile duct
	May be associated with ascending cholangitis

Finding an enlarged common duct at the time of surgery is also an indication for IOC. Gallstones obstructing the pancreatic duct are frequently a cause of pancreatitis. After pancreatitis resolves, interval cholecystectomy should be performed (Table 18-1).

Chapter 19

Pancreas

Acute Pancreatitis

Acute pancreatitis usually is a **nonbacterial inflammation** of the pancreas caused by activation, interstitial liberation, and the digestion of the gland by its own enzymes. It is characterized clinically by acute abdominal pain, elevated concentrations of pancreatic enzymes in blood, and an increase in the amount of pancreatic enzyme in the urine. In the United States, the most common cause of acute pancreatitis is **cholelithiasis**.

During a mild attack, the morphologic changes are characterized by pancreatic and peripancreatic edema and fat necrosis, but pancreatic necrosis is absent. This often is referred to as **edematous pancreatitis**. This mild form may become severe (or it may be severe from the onset); in its severe form, extensive pancreatic and peripancreatic fat necrosis, pancreatic parenchymal necrosis, and hemorrhage into and around the pancreas is evident. This form of disease is referred to as **hemorrhagic** or **necrotizing pancreatitis**. During an episode of acute inflammation, both exocrine and endocrine functions of the gland are impaired for weeks or months. If the cause (cholelithiasis) and any complications (pseudocyst) are eliminated, the pancreas usually returns to normal. Acute pancreatitis, even multiple attacks of acute pancreatitis, rarely lead to chronic pancreatitis.

Management of Acute Pancreatitis

The treatment of uncomplicated acute pancreatitis is medical and is directed primarily toward the restoration of fluid and electrolyte balance and avoidance of secretory stimulation of the pancreas. Complications of acute pancreatitis include adult respiratory distress syndrome (ARDS), pseudocyst, infected pancreatic necrosis, and pancreatic or peripancreatic abscess. Surgical intervention in the management of acute pancreatitis is reserved for patients who develop those complications previously noted.

In acute pancreatitis a diverse spectrum of illness is seen, varying from a mild, short-lived, self-limited disease to a severe toxic condition associated with shock, hypovolemia, multiple medical derangements, and ultimately death. The clinical presentation alone may be quite suggestive of the diagnosis. The predominant clinical feature of acute pancreatitis is **abdominal pain**. The pain normally begins in the **epigastrium**, achieving maximal intensity several hours into the illness. In most patients, the pain has a penetrating quality, radiating to the back. In patients with **alcohol-induced pancreatitis**, the pain often commences 12 to 48 hours after an episode of inebriation. In contrast, patients with gallstone pancreatitis typically experience the pain after a large meal.

Typical findings on physical examination include tachycardia, fever, epigastric tenderness, and abdominal distension. Abdominal distension may be the result of a paralytic ileus arising from the retroperitoneal irritation or it may be secondary to a retroperitoneal phlegmon. **Severe pancreatitis associated with hemorrhage** into the retroperitoneum may produce two distinctive physical signs: **Turner's sign** (bluish discoloration of the flank) or **Cullen's sign** (bluish discoloration around the umbilicus). These signs are seen in less than 3% of patients with pancreatitis and result from the tracking of blood-stained fluid through the tissue planes of the abdominal wall to the flank or along the falciform ligament to the umbilical region.

The diagnosis is often suspected on the basis of clinical presentation and is supported by finding **elevated amylase and/or lipase levels**. Clinical and laboratory evidence of pancreatitis can be supported by radiographic procedures. Currently, computed tomography (CT) is the most widely accepted and sensitive method used to confirm the diagnosis of pancreatitis. The clinical course of up to 90% of patients with acute pancreatitis follows a mild, self-limited course; in 10% to 15% of patients, however, a severe form of illness develops. It is possible to predict the severity of an attack of pancreatitis and the overall prognosis using routine available clinical and laboratory determinations. The most widely used predictive criteria involve 11 prognostic signs identified by **Ranson** in 1974 (Table 19-1).

Chronic Pancreatitis

Chronic pancreatitis is characterized clinically by recurrent, acute episodes of abdominal pain indistinguishable from those of acute pancreatitis. Diabetes and exocrine insufficiency occur as the disease progresses. In the United States, the most common cause of chronic pancreatitis is **alcoholism**. Morphologically, chronic pancreatitis is characterized by a permanent and usually progressive destruction of pancreatic parenchyma. The acinar cells are destroyed first, replaced by dense fibrosis. In chronic pancreatitis, unlike acute pancreatitis, the morphologic changes are irreversible and progressive, even if the cause (e.g., alcoholism) is removed. Management of

TABLE 19-1.

Ranson's Early Prognostic Signs of Acute Pancreatitis

At Admission	During Initial 48 Hours
Age > 55	Hematocrit fall > 10%
WBC > 16,000 cells/ mm^3	BUN elevation > 5 mg/dL
Serum LDH > 350 IU/L	Serum Ca^{2+} fall to < 8 mg/dL
SGOT > 250 U/dL	Pao$_2$ < 60 mm Hg
Blood glucose > 200 mg/dL	Base deficit > 4 mEq/L
	Estimated fluid sequestration > 6 L

Number of Criteria	Mortality
0–2	Essentially no mortality
3–4	15%
	Half require ICU admission
5–6	50%
	Almost all require ICU admission
> 7	> 50%

acute exacerbations of chronic pancreatitis is similar to the management of acute pancreatitis. Surgical intervention for relief of chronic pain is possible, but it is impossible to state in precise terms.

PANCREATIC CYSTS

Three types of pancreatic cysts occur: (1) congenital, (2) pseudocysts, and (3) neoplastic. Of these, pseudocysts are the most common. Congenital cysts are of little clinical importance except when they are multiple and part of the systemic disease cystic fibrosis.

Pseudocysts are localized collections of fluid with high concentrations of pancreatic enzymes; they usually occur as a complication of pancreatitis. They are located either within the parenchyma or in one of the potential spaces that separate the gland from the adjacent abdominal viscera. They usually are found in the lesser sac behind the stomach. If mature pseudocysts are less than 5 cm in diameter, they may not require treatment but should be followed by serial ultrasound. Cysts requiring surgical intervention are usually drained internally, although external drainage and excision are other options. A portion of the wall should always be biopsied to exclude a diagnosis of cystadenocarcinoma of the pancreas.

PANCREATIC CARCINOMA

In the United States, cancer of the exocrine pancreas is the fourth leading cause of death in men and the fifth in women. At the time of diagnosis, the tumor is confined to the pancreas in fewer than 10% of patients, and in **75% of cases**, pancreatic cancer occurs in the **head of the pancreas**. Approximately 75% of patients with pancreatic head carcinoma present with obstructive jaundice, weight loss (average of 20 pounds), and deep-seated abdominal pain.

A CT scan should be done after baseline laboratory studies confirm an elevated bilirubin. A dynamic CT scan with fine cuts through the head of the pancreas often defines a mass in the head of the pancreas. Evidence of metastatic spread or involvement of the superior mesenteric artery may be noted; these two features deem the patient unresectable. Fine-needle aspiration (FNA) can be performed for accurate tissue diagnosis in patients who are not candidates for surgery.

Endoscopic retrograde cholangiopancreatography (**ERCP**) is indicated for the relief of biliary obstruction for carcinomas that are not resectable, or if a definite mass is not seen on CT scan. In those patients determined preoperatively to be resectable, pancreatoduodenectomy (**Whipple resection**) is the most commonly performed surgery for carcinoma of the pancreatic head. Surgical palliation in patients with unresectable pancreatic carcinoma is directed toward relief of obstructive jaundice, gastric outlet obstruction, and pain.

ISLET CELL NEOPLASMS

Insulinoma

These tumors arise from beta cells and are the most common islet cell neoplasms. The classic diagnostic criteria (**Whipple's triad**) are usually present: (1) hypoglycemic symptoms produced by fasting, (2) blood glucose concentrations less than 50 mg/dL during symptomatic episodes, and (3) relief of symptoms during intravenous administration of glucose. The most useful diagnostic test is the demonstration of fasting hypoglycemia with inappropriately high serum levels of insulin. A ratio of plasma insulin to glucose of greater than 0.3 is diagnostic. Treatment consists of removal of the adenoma. Surreptitious self-administration of insulin may mimic this tumor. Circulating C-peptide levels are normal in these patients but are elevated in patients with insulinoma.

Gastrinoma (Zollinger-Ellison Syndrome)

The principal manifestation of Zollinger-Ellison syndrome (ZES) is due to gastric acid hypersecretion caused by excessive gastrin production by the tumor. Although the normal pancreas does not contain gastrin-producing cells, most gastrinomas arise in the pancreas. Other gastrinomas are found chiefly in the duodenum. One-fourth of gastrinomas are associated with multiple endocrine neoplasia type I (MEN-I) syndrome, in which the tumors are usually multiple and benign; those without MEN-I (sporadic gastrinomas) are more often single and malignant.

Symptoms of gastrinomas are those of gastric acid hypersecretion: severe refractory peptic ulcer disease and diarrhea (resulting from fat malabsorption as massive quantities of acid destroy pancreatic lipase). The diagnosis of gastrinoma requires the demonstration of fasting hypergastrinemia (greater than 200 pg/mL) in the presence of gastric acid hypersecretion. A paradoxical **increase** in **serum gastrin levels** in response to intravenously administered secretin (**secretin stimulation test**) confirms the diagnosis. The medical management of gastrinomas is treatment with hydrogen potassium proton pump inhibitor. In patients with MEN-I, the tumors are multiple and generally unresectable. All patients with **sporadic gastrinoma** should undergo **surgical exploration** unless there is evidence of extensive metastatic disease.

Chapter 20

Spleen

The spleen is the second largest organ of the reticuloendothelial system. It is located in the posterior left upper abdomen, where its relationships to the diaphragm, stomach, pancreas, left kidney, and splenic flexure of the colon are maintained by suspensory ligaments. The normal adult spleen is slightly concave, solid, dark red, and measures $3 \times 8 \times 14$ cm, with a mass of 100 to 150 g. During early fetal development, the spleen produces red and white blood cells. By the fifth month of fetal development, the spleen and other extramedullary sites of blood cell production no longer have hematopoietic function, but they retain the capacity for life. The spleen is a sophisticated filter with blood cell monitoring and management functions and important immune functions. When the spleen is removed, these functions are lost.

INDICATIONS FOR SURGERY

Aside from trauma, from a surgical standpoint, **splenectomy** is indicated in two broad categories: (1) to control or stage disease and (2) for chronic or severe hypersplenism (Table 20-1). With trauma, the spleen is the most frequently injured intraabdominal organ. With associated injuries, mortality rates approaching 10% are noted with splenic rupture. Splenectomy is usually indicated in adults with a severely injured spleen, but in children splenic salvage has been advocated. This is based largely on the preservation of the spleen's important role in cellular and humoral immunity.

OVERWHELMING POSTSPLENECTOMY INFECTION (OPSI)

Asplenic patients have increased susceptibility to developing overwhelming infections characterized by fulminant bacteremia, menin-

SURGERY

TABLE 20-1.

Indications for Splenectomy

To Control or Stage Basic Disease

Hereditary spherocytosis

Autoimmune anemia

Hodgkin's disease

Ruptured spleen

Immune thrombocytopenic purpura (ITP)

Thrombotic thrombocytopenic purpura (TTP)

Primary tumors or cysts

For Chronic or Severe Hypersplenism

Hairy cell leukemia

Lymphoproliferative disorders (non-Hodgkin's lymphoma, chronic lymphocyte leukemia)

Felty's syndrome

Agnogenic myeloid metaplasia

Thalassemia major

Gaucher's disease

Hemodialysis splenomegaly

Splenic vein thrombosis

Sickle cell disease

Acquired immunodeficiency syndrome (AIDS)

Thrombocytopenia associated with drug abuse

gitis, or pneumonia. Following splenectomy, the risk of overwhelming infections is approximately 60 times greater than normal, and may be as high as 0.5% to 1.9% yearly. The **risk is greatest in children younger than 4 years of age within 2 years of splenectomy** (80% of cases). Common offending organisms include *Streptococcus pneumoniae, Neisseria meningitidis, Escherichia coli,* and *Haemophilus influenzae. S. pneumoniae* accounts for more than 50% of cases.

Antibiotic prophylaxis or early antibiotic therapy may be effective in reducing the incidence of OPSI. Because 50% of patients develop sepsis from *S. pneumoniae,* penicillin can be administered prophylactically or immediately following the onset of a febrile upper respiratory tract infection. Immunization with Pneumovax and vaccines against *H. influenzae* should ideally be administered 2 to 3 weeks before splenectomy.

Chapter 21

Liver

ANATOMY

Historically, concepts of hepatobiliary anatomy developed from initial misinterpretations of ligamentous reflections of the peritoneum (mainly the falciform ligament) and its division of the "right" and "left" lobes of the liver. The topographic right and left lobes are the portions of the liver on the respective side of the falciform ligament. The caudate (Spigelian) lobe is delineated by the posterior (transverse) extension of the falciform ligament (ligamentum venosum—the remnant of the ductus venosus) on the left, and the impression of the inferior vena cava on the right. The quadrate lobe is anterior to the caudate lobe and is bound by the gallbladder fossa on the right, the groove of falciform ligament to the left, and posteriorly by the porta hepatis (umbilical fissure). Unfortunately, this topographic anatomy bears faint resemblance to the true anatomy of the liver. The lobar anatomy, as defined by the distribution of the major branches of the portal vein, is best demonstrated by direct injection of the left and right portal veins. This demonstrates that the right and left lobes of the liver are delineated by a line (**Cantlie's line**) passing through the fossa of the gallbladder and to the left of the inferior vena cava (Fig. 21-1).

LIVER FUNCTION

The liver is an important **liaison between the digestive system and other areas of the body**. Specifically, these features include: (1) a dual blood supply; (2) a deliberate architectural arrangement of single cells and cell masses, which facilitates exchange between blood and hepatocytes; (3) orientation of the hepatocytes, which separates biliary and blood flow; and (4) an organized biliary excretory system, which regulates the enterohepatic circulation. The liver receives blood from the arterial and portal circulation, processes nu-

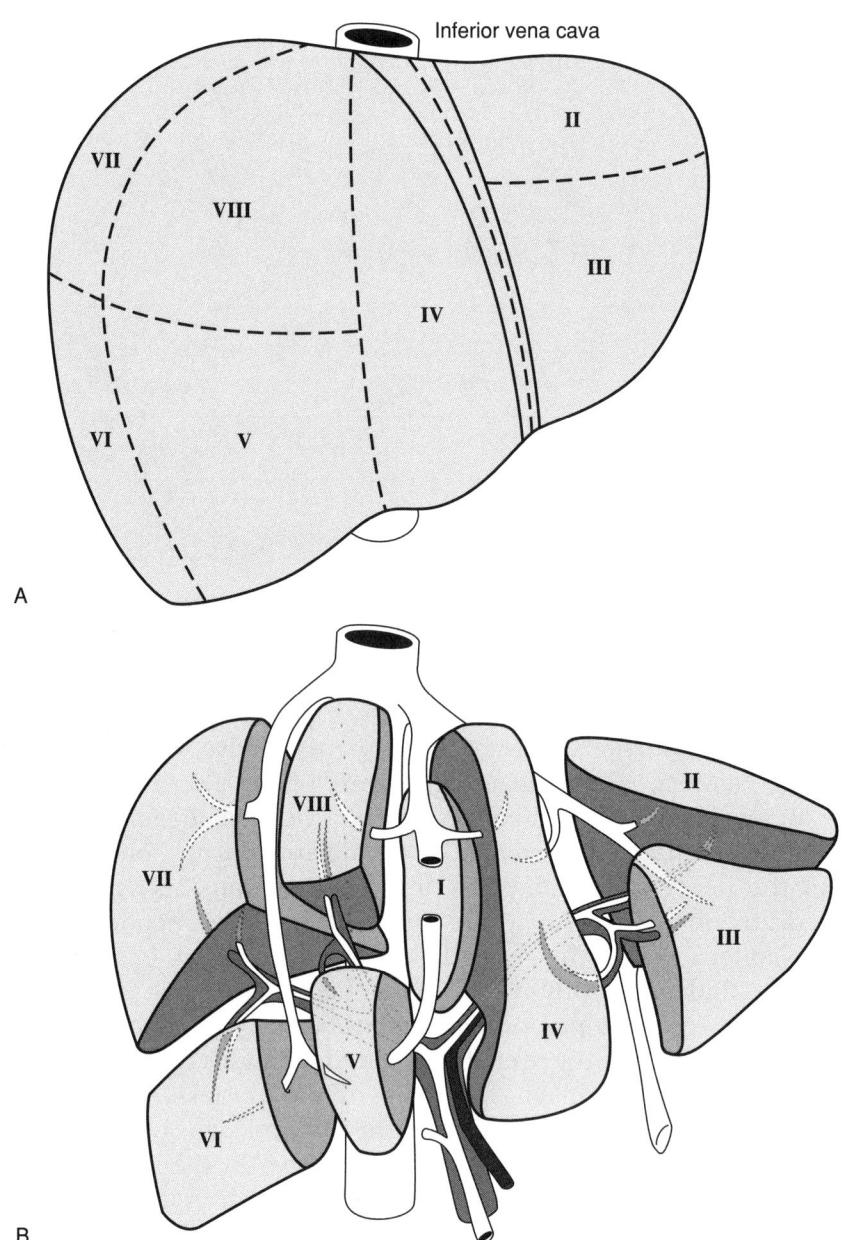

Figure 21-1.
Segmental anatomy of the liver as defined by Couinaud. *A*, Intact liver;
B, schematic representation.

trients and metabolized toxins and wastes, and stores, transforms, and distributes them to the vascular, biliary, or lymphatic circulations. To accomplish this, the liver expends approximately 20% of the body's energy and consumes 20% to 25% of the total oxygen utilized, quantities that are more impressive when recalling that the liver represents only 4% to 5% of total body mass. Mean total hepatic blood flow has been estimated to be approximately 100 to 130 mL/kg/min. Approximately 70% to 75% of total hepatic blood flow comes from the portal vein, whereas the remainder comes from the hepatic artery. Changes in liver homeostasis are readily reflected by measurement of "liver functions." Table 21-1 outlines many of the common tests and their significance.

HEPATIC RESECTION

The indications for hepatic resection include (1) trauma with resultant devascularization of hepatic tissue, (2) cysts, (3) granulomas,

TABLE 21-1.
Laboratory Tests in Liver Disease

Laboratory Test	Change in Liver Disease	Significance of Change in Liver Disease
ALT	Increase	Correlates with hepatic cell death
AST	Increase	Correlates with hepatic cell death
ALP	Increase	Biliary duct obstruction
		Liver tumor; metastatic liver tumor
		Note: normally increased during growth and pregnancy
		increased in bone tumors
		heat stability/electrophoresis can distinguish isoenzyme
		increased 5′N, LAP, GGT with ALP suggestive of biliary disease
GGT	Increase	Extrahepatic biliary obstruction
		Note: increased in chronic alcoholics
		increased in myocardial infarction, neuromuscular disease
		useful in following alcohol consumption
LAP	Increase	Cholestasis
		Note: increased in pregnancy
		ubiquitous enzyme
5′-N	Increase	Cholestasis
Albumin	Decrease	Chronically impaired liver function
		Note: dependent on nutritional status of patient
		decreased in conditions associated with loss/consumption:
		nephrotic syndrome
		protein losing enteropathy
		sepsis
		burns
		need adequate thyroid and adrenal function
Transferrin	Decrease	Reflects more acute changes in liver function and nutritional status

ALT: alanine aminotransferase; AST: aspartate aminotransferase; ALP: alkaline phosphatase; GGT: gamma glutamyl transferase; LAP: leucine aminopeptidase; 5′-N: 5 prime nucleotidase.

(4) primary neoplasms of the liver, and (5) secondary malignant tumors that involve the liver either by direct extension or as metastatic lesions. Removal of up to 75% of the liver is compatible with life. Following excision of this amount, patients maintain normal capacity for liver metabolic and synthetic activity. **Regeneration** results from significant hypertrophy of the remaining tissue. The remaining portion of the liver responds rapidly after the initial result, and regeneration usually restores the liver to its original mass within 6 weeks after resection. A cirrhotic liver, however, has very little capacity for regeneration.

PORTAL HYPERTENSION

There are no venous valves in the portal vein. This has several important implications and consequences: (1) portal hypertension is reflected through all the portal tributaries; (2) the portal vein has low resistance and high flow, despite much of the loss of kinetic energy in the digestive tract capillary network; and (3) the architecture of the liver must accommodate both the high-pressure arterial system and the low-pressure portal system. From a surgical standpoint, the most important factor above is the consequence of portal hypertension and manifestations of increased collateral flow through the portosystemic communications (Fig. 21-2).

PORTOSYSTEMIC ANASTOMOSES

The most important natural portosystemic anastomoses include the following.

1. The **left gastric or coronary vein**, which joins the splenic or portal vein near its confluence and connects with the esophageal venous plexus and also with tributaries of the superior vena cava. This often is the most important anastomotic system in the development of esophageal varices.
2. The **short gastric and left gastroepiploic veins**, which connect to the splenic vein and contribute to the formation of gastric and esophageal varices.
3. The **umbilical and periumbilical veins**. This venous system is usually atrophied in the adult but may remain patent connecting the superficial venous system to the portal system, particularly in cirrhotic patients. Physical findings associated with this are the continuous venous hum over the liver, in the epigastrium (Cruveilhier-Baumgarten sign), and **caput medusae**.

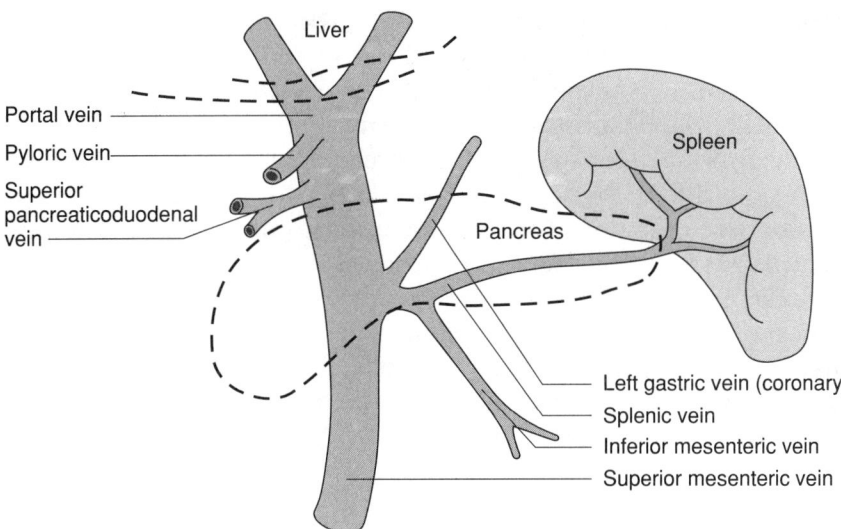

Figure 21-2.
Portosystemic collateral pathways.

4. **Tributaries of the inferior mesenteric vein**, which include the superior hemorrhoidal veins, which communicate with the middle and inferior hemorrhoidal veins of the systemic system and may cause large hemorrhoids.

5. Other **retroperitoneal communications** such as connections to renal and adrenal veins. In conditions in which there is altered portal blood flow, increased blood is shunted through these naturally occurring portosystemic shunts.

Increased pressure in the portal circulation may result from prehepatic (thrombosis of the portal vein), intrahepatic (cirrhosis), or posthepatic (obstruction of the hepatic veins—**Budd-Chiari syndrome**) portal venous obstruction. Naturally occurring collateral venous channels between the portal circulation and the inferior vena cava form nature's efforts to bypass the obstructive flow. Peptic erosion or rupture of the collateral veins in the esophagus gives rise to serious **gastrointestinal bleeding**, with death following rapidly if the hemorrhage is not controlled.

MANAGEMENT OF PORTAL HYPERTENSION

Emergency treatment consists of **intravenous fluid resuscitation** and control of hemorrhage with **balloon tamponade**. Intravenous **vasopressin** may decrease bleeding. Definitive treatment consists of sclerotherapy or rubberband ligation of bleeding varices. **Intractable bleeding** is managed with the **transcutaneous intra-**

hepatic portosystemic shunt (TIPS) procedure where available. Otherwise, emergency shunt operation should be performed.

With the advent of the minimally invasive techniques described above, the role of surgical management of portal hypertension and esophageal bleeding has been reserved for those patients who do not respond to medical management. Central shunts, or those created between the portal circulation and the inferior vena cava (portacaval, interposition PTFE "H" portacaval shunt, mesocaval shunt, or interposition PTFE "C" mesocaval shunt), have a higher incidence of encephalopathy (30%). Selective shunts (Warren shunt or distal splenorenal shunt) have a lower incidence of encephalopathy (10%) but are contraindicated in patients with ascites. They are used infrequently in an emergency.

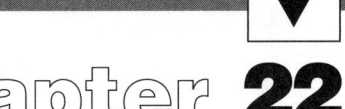

Chapter 22

Intestines

Intestinal obstruction is present when an interference occurs with the normal passage of intestinal contents. Such obstruction may result from extraluminal (adhesions), intraluminal (bezoar, gallstones), or intramural (Crohn's disease, tumors) obstructions. The term *mechanical bowel obstruction* is used to describe an actual physical barrier, whereas *ileus* denotes a functional failure of progressive intestinal transit. **Simple obstruction** refers to an obstructed lumen with an intact blood supply. If the mesenteric vessels are occluded, then **strangulated obstruction** is present. **Closed loop obstruction** results when both loops of the bowel are obstructed. Obstructions are additionally classified as partial or complete, acute or chronic, high or low, and colonic versus small intestinal. The most common cause of small bowel obstruction is **postoperative adhesions** (65% to 80%), hernias (15% to 25%), and malignant tumors (10% to 15%). Colonic obstruction usually arises from cancer (60%), diverticulitis (15%), or volvulus (15%).

Signs and Symptoms

The four cardinal symptoms and signs of intestinal obstruction are (1) crampy, episodic abdominal **pain**, (2) **vomiting**, (3) **obstipation**, and (4) abdominal **distension** (Fig. 22-1). Ileus usually is not painful, except for generalized discomfort from distension. Reflexive vomiting occurs almost immediately after the onset of obstruction; however, it is unusual in colonic obstruction, except for volvulus. Abdominal distension is a late finding and may be absent in high small bowel obstruction if vomiting occurs and decompresses the intestine.

Diagnosis

The initial blood studies may reveal mild to moderate dehydration. The **abdominal and chest radiographs** usually are the most

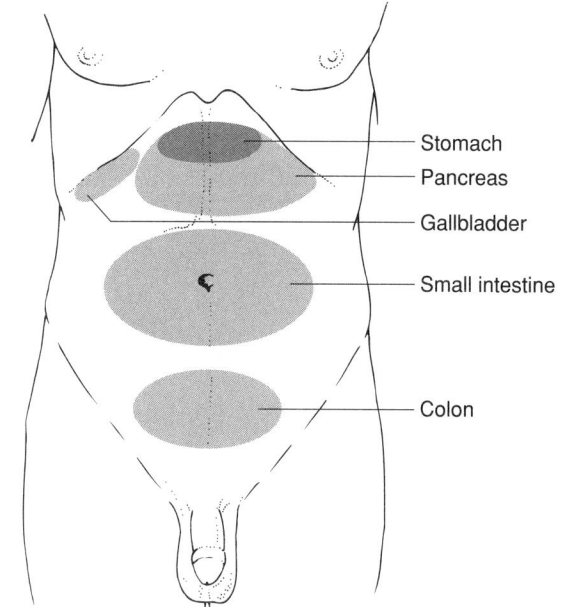

Figure 22-1.
Pain from intra-abdominal viscera.

Stomach
Pancreas
Gallbladder
Small intestine
Colon

important diagnostic tests and should be performed early in the patient's evaluation. Demonstration of air-fluid levels on an upright or decubitus abdominal film is of diagnostic significance. A **barium enema** in patients without evidence of previous surgery (adhesions) or no evidence of hernia is important to evaluate the possibility of colonic tumor or volvulus. The use of barium in either a small bowel series or an enteroclysis study can distinguish adynamic ileus from partial or complete bowel obstruction. In patients with ileus, barium requires 4 to 6 hours to reach the colon; mechanical obstruction produces dilated bowel and progression of the barium to the site of obstruction in 1 hour or less.

Management

The principles of management of intestinal obstruction are fluid and electrolyte therapy, decompression of the gastrointestinal tract with an indwelling tube, and timely surgical intervention. The differentiation between partial and complete small bowel obstruction is important because less than 20% of patients with partial obstruction require surgical intervention.

APPENDICITIS

Acute appendicitis is the most common acute surgical condition of the abdomen. The disease occurs in all ages but is most common in the second and third decades of life. Obstruction of the lumen of the appendix causes a **closed loop obstruction**, with continued normal se-

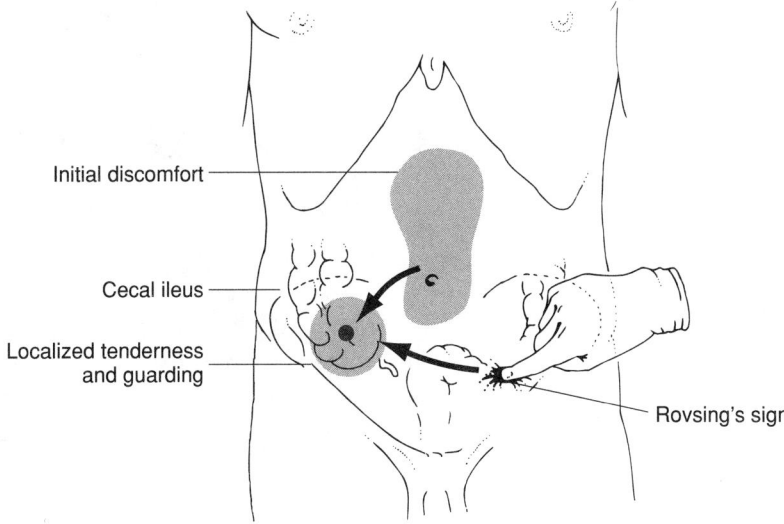

Figure 22-2.
Some physical signs of appendicitis before rupture.

cretion of the appendiceal mucosa together with bacterial overgrowth rapidly producing distension. **Abdominal pain** is the prime symptom of acute appendicitis. Classically, the pain is initially periumbilical; after 4 to 6 hours, the pain localizes in the **right lower quadrant**. Anorexia usually accompanies acute appendicitis.

On physical examination, a patient may have a low-grade fever and the pain is well localized in the right lower quadrant. When the appendix lies in the pelvis, tenderness on rectal examination is noted. The leukocyte count is usually elevated. **Appendectomy** is the treatment of choice (Fig. 22-2).

TUMORS OF THE INTESTINES

Polyposis of the Intestinal Tract

Familial polyposis is a disease characterized by multiple polyps of the colon and rectum. It is inherited as a Mendelian dominant condition. The polyps usually appear at puberty. The most serious complication is **malignant transformation** of the polyps. Most patients with untreated colon cancer die before the age of 50 years. Treatment consists of proctocolectomy and ileoanal pull-through, abdominal colectomy and ileoproctostomy, or proctocolectomy and ileostomy.

Gardner's syndrome is a variant of familial polyposis and is also inherited as a Mendelian dominant condition. It is associated with osteomas of the skull, multiple sebaceous cysts of the scalp, and desmoid tumors. It involves both the small and large intestines.

These polyps also undergo **malignant transformation**; management is the same as that described for familial polyposis.

Peutz-Jeghers Syndrome

Peutz-Jeghers syndrome is a familial disease in which there is an association between hamartomatous polyps of the gastrointestinal tract and pigmented spots on the lips, buccal mucosa, and hands. These polyps **do not undergo malignant change**. The small intestine contains more polyps than any other portion of the intestinal tract, but the entire tract is involved. Symptoms arise from intussusception, which may spontaneously reduce or progress to intestinal obstruction.

MALIGNANT TUMORS OF THE SMALL INTESTINE

Cancer of the small intestine is **rare**. It is manifested by bleeding, obstruction, or both. Adenocarcinoma tends to encircle and obstruct the bowel. Smooth muscle tumors are bulky and polypoid with central ulceration, which gives rise to bleeding. **Carcinoid tumors** in the small intestine metastasize with greater frequency than carcinoids elsewhere in the gastrointestinal tract. Carcinoid tumors that metastasize to the liver are capable of producing **carcinoid syndrome**, a complex of symptoms consisting of episodic flushing of the skin, abdominal cramps, diarrhea, and asthma. These symptoms are caused by the **excessive levels of serotonin** released by the tumor into the systemic circulation. Benign nonfunctioning carcinoid tumors occur primarily in the appendix.

The diagnosis of functioning carcinoid tumor is made by the detection of **increased hydroxyindoleacetic acid (5-HIAA) in the urine**—a breakdown product of serotonin metabolism. Treatment requires resection of the entire tumor, which is rarely possible. However, even when known tumor is left behind, symptoms may be relieved by drug treatment.

CARCINOMA OF THE COLON AND RECTUM

The large intestine is a frequent site of carcinoma. The type of lesion and the symptomatology differ greatly on the two sides of the colon. In the **left colon**, a constricting **napkin-ring–like lesion** is found. Associated with it are symptoms of mechanical obstruction (including alternating constipation and diarrhea), crampy abdominal pain, and distension of the bowel. Blood may be noticed in the stool, and sometimes there is an alteration in the caliber of the stools.

In the right colon, the lesions are often bulky and cauliflowerlike and are less likely to encircle the bowel. In addition, the liquid character of the fecal material on this side of the colon diminishes the likelihood of obstructive symptoms. **Right-sided lesions** have a greater propensity for blood loss, and a profound anemia can develop. Patients may present with fatigue or exacerbations of lung and heart disease as a result of anemia. Carcinoma of the rectum presents with symptoms that resemble those of carcinoma of the left colon. **Carcinoma of the rectum and sigmoid** comprise the largest percentage of neoplasms in the large bowel.

Diagnosis and Treatment

The diagnosis is often suspected on history, and physical examination may reveal a palpable mass on rectal examination or occult blood in the stool. Further evaluation by sigmoidoscopy and barium enema or by colonoscopy should be undertaken. Colonoscopy allows for biopsy and resection of smaller polyps.

When a diagnosis of **colonic or rectal carcinoma** has been made, **surgical resection** should be undertaken. The prognosis depends on stage of the disease at the time of resection. The Astler and Coller modification of Dukes' classification in the staging system is generally used: stage A, invasion to the muscularis; stage B1, invasion to the serosa; stage B2, invasion of the pericolonic fat; stage C1, invasion to the serosa with lymph node metastases; stage C2, invasion of the pericolonic fat and lymph node metastases; and stage D, metastatic disease (Table 22-1).

TABLE 22-1.

Dukes' Classification of Colon Cancer

Stage	Criteria
A	Invasion to the muscularis mucosa
B1	Invasion to the serosa
B2	Invasion to the pericolonic fat
C1	Invasion to the serosa with lymph node involvement
C2	Invasion to the pericolonic fat with lymph node involvement
D	Metastatic disease

Currently, for **Dukes' stage C colon cancer and stage B or greater rectal cancer, postoperative chemoradiation** is recommended.

DIVERTICULAR DISEASE OF THE COLON

Diverticular disease and diverticulosis are terms used to indicate the presence of colonic diverticula, a condition that is rare before the age of 30 years but becomes more common with increasing age. Diverticulosis appears to be a phenomena of the industrial revolution and Western society. In general, it is believed that the diverticula are formed by increased colonic pressure, which forces the mucosa through weak points in the colonic wall. The transmural pressure is greatest in the sigmoid, which is the predominant location of diverticula. The **diverticula** are predominantly located on the **mesenteric side of the antimesenteric tenia** (Fig. 22-3).

Diverticular disease is complicated by infection or hemorrhage, and either of these may be an indication for surgery. **Diverticulitis** denotes **infection** associated with diverticula. The term is somewhat of a misnomer because the infectious process commonly associated with diverticular disease is pericolonic in nature and predominantly involves the surrounding soft tissues. The infection is the result of a perforation of a diverticulum, leading to extravasa-

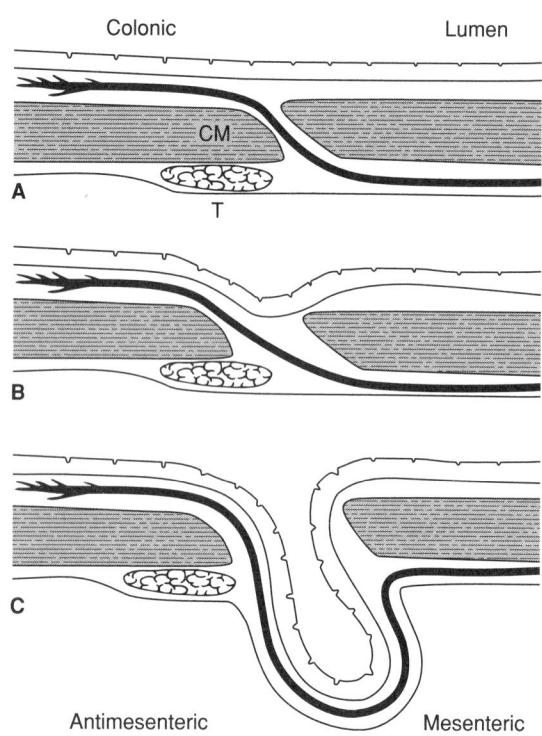

Figure 22-3.
The relation of a diverticulum to mural vasculature. *A,* The vasa recta penetrate the colonic wall obliquely at specific sites in the circular muscle (CM), usually along the mesenteric side of the teniae (T). *B,* As the diverticulum begins to herniate through the colonic wall, the blood vessels are drawn along. *C,* The vasa recta eventually become draped over the dome of the diverticulum and are prone to rupture after injury arising within the lumen of the colon.

tion of feces. This can be minimal and cause a localized confined process, or it can be significant, resulting in **abscess** formation or even generalized **peritonitis**.

Management of Diverticular Disease

Patients with acute diverticulitis usually complain of **pain** in the **left lower abdomen**. Computed tomography (CT) scan is the diagnostic technique of choice used to confirm the suspected diagnosis of diverticulitis. If an abscess is present, CT-guided drainage may be used. Oral **antibiotics** (for mild cases) or intravenous antibiotics (for more aggressive cases) are the treatment of choice. Seventy percent of patients who recover from an uncomplicated episode of diverticulitis have no recurrence.

In patients whose conditions are toxic, with generalized peritonitis, **surgical resection with colostomy** may be necessary. Patients who have recovered from two or more episodes of diverticulitis or patients with evidence of **fistula** (bladder, vagina, small intestine, skin) should undergo elective **repair and sigmoid resection**.

Colonic diverticula are formed where the colonic arterioles penetrate the muscle wall of the bowel; thus, there is an intimate association between arteriole and the diverticulum. These vessels are prone to disrupt, leading to **hemorrhage**.

Management of massive bleeding from the lower gastrointestinal tract requires **intravascular resuscitation with transfusion**, and a nasogastric tube should be placed and aspirated to exclude an upper gastrointestinal source of the bleeding. Proctoscopy should also be performed to exclude an anorectal cause of bleeding. Nuclear scan with radiolabeled red blood cells is recommended to localize the bleeding and, once localized, arteriography with embolization or intraarterial vasopressin can be attempted. Colonic bleeding ceases spontaneously in 85% of cases. Surgical exploration for an unidentified source of gastrointestinal bleeding is not recommended and carries a mortality rate of 20% to 40%.

INFLAMMATORY BOWEL DISEASE

The term inflammatory bowel disease encompasses two major entities: ulcerative colitis and Crohn's disease. **Ulcerative colitis** (UC) is an inflammatory process involving the colonic mucosa, characterized by alterations in bowel function and symptoms of intestinal inflammation. It is limited to the **colon and rectum**. The most frequent sign of UC is hematochezia, the passage of bright red blood from the rectum. Tenesmus and diarrhea are also frequent symptoms. **Crohn's disease**, or regional enteritis, can occur anywhere in the **intestinal tract from the mouth to the anus**. Crohn's disease and UC appear closely related when the disease exists in the colon, and 15% of cases cannot be clearly distinguished. The differentiation of the two is of therapeutic significance in that there is significant recurrence of disease in the small intestine in patients with Crohn's disease treated by colectomy. Crohn's disease has transmural microscopic involvement; the disease is limited to the mucosa in UC. Features most useful in distinguishing UC from Crohn's disease are listed in Table 22-2.

Management

Indications for surgery in **UC** include active bleeding unresponsive to medical therapy, risk of cancer, toxic megacolon, and severe bleeding. Because only the large intestine is involved, **proctocolectomy** should cure the patient of intestinal disease. The patient at risk for cancer is one who has had total colonic involvement for more than 10 years. Surgical management of **Crohn's disease** is limited to the complications of the disease. Usually this involves **resection of the diseased segment of the intestine responsible for the complications**, including internal fistulas and abscesses, intestinal obstruction, perianal fistulas, toxic megacolon, and poor response to medical therapy. Recurrent disease is not reduced by obtaining a wide margin of uninvolved intestine.

TABLE 22-2.

Inflammatory Disease of the Colon

	Ulcerative Colitis	Crohn's Disease
Usual involvement	Rectum, left colon	Anywhere
Rectal bleeding	Common, continuous	Uncommon, intermittent
Rectal involvement	Almost always	Approximately 50%
Fistulas	Rare	Common
Ulcers	Shaggy, irregular, continuous	Linear, transverse fissures
Bowel stricture	Rare	Common
Carcinoma	Increases incidence	Slight increased incidence
Toxic megacolon	Occurs in both diseases	

ANORECTAL DISEASE

Hemorrhoids

Hemorrhoids are found at the distal end of the rectum within the anal canal. Internal hemorrhoids are above the dentate line, and external hemorrhoids are the vascular complexes under the anoderm of the anal canal.

Internal hemorrhoids, which are covered by mucosa, typically bleed and prolapse but do not cause pain. Internal hemorrhoids can be classified as follows: first-degree hemorrhoids, which bleed; second-degree hemorrhoids, which bleed and prolapse; third-degree hemorrhoids, which bleed and prolapse and require manual reduction; and fourth-degree hemorrhoids, which bleed and incarcerate and cannot be reduced. Prolapsed and thrombosed hemorrhoids can induce intense anal spasm and be quite painful.

Management of Hemorrhoids

Conservative measures such as increasing dietary fiber and fluid intake, reducing narcotic analgesia, and decreasing alcohol intake usually control first- and second-degree hemorrhoids. Elastic ligation is an effective treatment for third-degree hemorrhoids. The excision of hemorrhoids should be limited to large third- and fourth-degree hemorrhoids. Patients seen in the emergency department with painful, acutely thrombosed external hemorrhoids should have excision performed under local anesthesia. Merely incising the hemorrhoid and expressing the clot carries a significant risk of recurrence of thrombosis. If the thrombosis has occurred more than 48 hours previously, conservative management with warm soaks is the preferred therapy.

Anal Fissure or Anal Ulcer

An anal fissure is a split in either the posterior or anterior midline just distal to the dentate line. Ninety percent are posterior. The characteristic symptoms of fissure or ulcer include tearing pain on defecation or blood on toilet paper or stool. The pain may continue for several hours after defecation. The cause is thought to be hard feces or prolonged diarrhea with stretching of the anal canal. When a fissure or ulcer is in an atypical location, Crohn's disease or tuberculosis should be suspected. Ninety percent of fissures or ulcers heal with use of stool softeners and local symptomatic care. For those patients requiring surgical intervention, lateral internal anal sphincterotomy is the procedure of choice.

HERNIA

A hernia is defined as a protrusion of a viscus through an opening in the wall of the cavity in which it is contained. Several terms are used to describe the various types of hernias. A **reducible** hernia is one in which the contents may be returned entirely to the cavity that ordinarily contains them. This is not possible in an **incarcerated** hernia. A painful acutely incarcerated hernia should be suspected of being strangulated until proven otherwise by early surgery. A strangulated hernia is one in which the blood supply of the viscus is impaired so that gangrene ultimately ensues.

Classification of Hernias

Hernias also are classified according to their location, with the most common type of hernia located in the **inguinal** region. Inguinal hernias are the most common hernias in both men and women. These can be either **direct** (herniation directly through the floor of the inguinal canal) or **indirect** (through the internal ring and along the spermatic cord). A **femoral** hernia passes through the femoral canal; therefore, the sac lies below the inguinal ligament. Femoral hernias are more common in women, but in absolute numbers. An **umbilical** hernia is a defect in the region of the umbilicus. A herniation occurring at the site of a previous surgery is called an **incisional** hernia. An **epigastric** hernia is a small nodular mass in the midline of the upper abdomen, which results from protrusion of the preperitoneal fat along the course of a vessel penetrating the linea alba. These hernias do not have a peritoneal sac.

Diagnosis and Treatment

The diagnosis of a hernia is made readily by the demonstration of a mass in one of the locations described. In all hernias, there is a risk of incarceration and strangulation, and surgical repair is recommended.

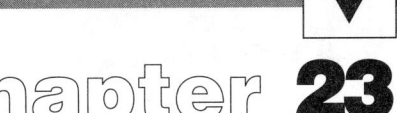

Adrenal Glands

Tumors of the adrenal medulla include **neuroblastomas** and **pheochromocytoma**. A pheochromocytoma is an endocrine tumor that produces norepinephrine and epinephrine. The chief symptom is sustained diastolic hypertension and paroxysmal hypertensive episodes. Ten percent of tumors arise in an extra-adrenal location, primarily in the paravertebral sympathetic chain. Ten percent are malignant, and 10% are bilateral. When these tumors are bilateral, they are likely to be familial. The diagnosis is based on increased urinary and plasma catecholamines. The tumor can be localized by computed tomography (CT), magnetic resonance imaging (MRI), or ^{131}I metaiodobenzaguanidine (MIBG) scanning. **Surgical resection** is the only curative procedure. Before surgery, the patient should be given drugs that prevent severe hypertension and catecholamine crisis.

TUMORS OF THE ADRENAL CORTEX

Tumors of the adrenal cortex result in a number of clinical syndromes, including Cushing's syndrome, Cushing's disease, and Conn's syndrome.

Cushing's Syndrome

Cushing's syndrome results from **hyperplasia** of the adrenal cortex. The typical signs of increased cortisol secretion are moon facies, buffalo hump, truncal obesity, wasting of extremities, and thinning of the skin. Treatment is surgical removal of the pituitary adenoma causing the adrenal hyperplasia.

Cushing's Disease

In Cushing's disease, the **increased cortisol levels** result from a functioning adenoma of the adrenal cortex. Removal of the adrenal tumor is the appropriate therapy.

Conn's Syndrome

Conn's syndrome, or **hyperaldosteronism**, is recognized clinically in patients with hypertension, muscular weakness, metabolic alkalosis, hypokalemia, suppressed plasma renin activity, and increased potassium and aldosterone excretion. These findings must be documented in the absence of diuretic therapy, chronic vomiting (or laxative abuse), or renal artery disease. Treatment is by excision of the involved adrenal.

Chapter 24

Urogenital System

Nephrolithiasis is a relatively common disorder affecting 1% to 3% of the adult population. History and physical examination, urinalysis, and plain film of the abdomen usually establish the diagnosis. More than 90% of stones within the urinary tract are radiopaque. **Intravenous pyelogram (IVP)** defines the relationship of the calculus to the pyelocalyceal system and the ureter. The exact location of the stones, presence of absence of obstruction, hydronephrosis, caliectasis, and renal/ureteric anomalies are all important information that can be determined by IVP. In the past, symptomatic stone removal required an open surgical procedure. Advances in fiberoptics with the subsequent development of small-caliber flexible instruments and extracorporeal shock wave lithotripsy (ESWL) has led to a decrease in open procedures.

BENIGN PROSTATIC HYPERTROPHY

Benign prostatic hypertrophy (BPH) is the most common disorder of the **prostate gland**. Although seldom life threatening, BPH can have significant impact on the quality of life. Hyperplastic growth of the prostate begins in men by the fifth decade. By the age of 80 years, almost 90% of men have histologic evidence of BPH. Men with clinically significant BPH have a group of symptoms termed **prostatism**. These symptoms include frequent urination and urgency, decreased force of the urine stream, hesitation in the initiation of flow, intermittency, a sensation of incomplete emptying, and nocturia to a variable degree. Patients presenting with these symptoms should undergo further evaluation. The best noninvasive test to evaluate prostatism is the flow of urine measured by an electronic device that calculates the velocity of urine flow. The maximal flow rate is normally 15 mL/sec. A reduction in the flow rate is suggestive of obstruction.

Men with only mild symptoms or asymptotic prostatic enlargement should be managed by watchful waiting, whereas those with urinary retention, recurrent infections, bladder stones, or renal insufficiency secondary to BPH should be treated surgically. **Transurethral resection of the prostate** (TURP) is the most common and most effective surgical procedure to treat BPH.

PROSTATIC INFECTIONS

Prostatic infections occur in a significant number of men and frequently require urologic attention. Infectious agents that may involve the prostate gland include the spectrum of gram-negative organisms, gram-positive cocci, gonococci, various mycotic organisms, *Mycobacterium* species, trichomonads, *Chlamydia* species, and *Candida* species. The ascending transurethral route of infection is usual, and exogenous infection is enhanced by urethral abnormalities. Hematogenous and descending spread of infection have been noted, especially with tuberculous prostatitis.

Suppurative acute prostatitis may be seen from pubescence throughout life. The organisms most frequently involved are gram-negative organisms, principally *Escherichia coli*. Acute gonococcal prostatitis is relatively uncommon. Symptoms include urgency, frequency, dysuria, perineal aching, rectal discomfort, and even chills and fever with bacteremia. Edema may predispose a patient to acute urinary tract infections. Urinalysis usually reveals pyuria, and the offending organism can often be cultured. Prostatic massage should be avoided to avert bacteremia. Therapy consists of vigorous **antibiotic therapy** based on culture and sensitivity results as well as bed rest, intermittent hot sitz baths, antipyretics, and restriction of sexual activity. Before antibiotic therapy, prostatic abscesses were frequent sequelae of acute prostatitis.

PROSTATE CARCINOMA

Carcinoma of the prostate is a very common neoplasm in older men. With the advent of the monoclonal antibody to detect elevations of **prostate-specific antigen (PSA)**, the detection rate has increased fourfold over the past decade. Additionally, ultrasound-guided biopsy of the prostate has improved diagnostic accuracy. An elevated serum acid phosphatase is characteristic of carcinoma of the prostate, whereas an elevated alkaline phosphatase is suggestive of bony disease. Treatment of **early carcinoma**, localized to the gland without extension beyond the capsule, is **total prosta-**

tectomy. External beam radiotherapy is an alternative method of treatment. Treatment of **advanced carcinoma** consists of **androgen blockade therapy** and/or **orchiectomy**. This treatment rapidly improves pain and anorexia and gradually relieves the obstructive urinary symptoms.

RENAL CELL CARCINOMA

Renal tumors account for approximately 2% of cancer deaths. There are three major types of malignant renal tumors, and renal cell carcinoma accounts for 85% of these lesions. There is often a tendency for the tumor to invade the venous system, extending into the vena cava and right heart. The classic triad of **pain, mass**, and **hematuria** occurs late and is seen in less than half of patients. **Erythrocythemia** is present in 2% of patients; erythropoietin has been extracted from these tumors. Hepatic cell dysfunction (**Stouffer's syndrome**), which is reversible with removal of the renal carcinoma, has been noted.

Early detection is often the result of abdominal imaging studies such as ultrasonography, computed tomography (CT) scan, and radioisotopic studies, which have been performed for evaluation of nonurologic studies. Metastases are demonstrated in one-third of patients at the time of diagnosis and include metastases to the lung, bone, lymph nodes, and skin. **Radical nephrectomy** with removal of ipsilateral adrenal and hilar nodes is the standard surgical procedure for resectable lesions.

LESIONS OF THE SCROTUM AND PENIS

Hydrocele

Hydrocele is a cystic enlargement of the **tunica vaginalis**. It may occur at any age and is frequently asymptomatic except for the presence of a mass. **Transillumination** usually confirms the diagnosis. Aspiration yields clear fluid. Repeated aspirations are of palliative value only; the procedure of choice is surgery, consisting of opening the sac and everting it about the testicle.

Varicocele

This condition is an undue **enlargement or varicosity of the pampiniform plexus**. Varicocele is more common on the **left side**.

Occasionally it is associated with a dragging, aching sensation in the testis on the involved side. The discomfort may be decreased with adequate support. On examination, the varicosity is evident along the structures of the cord above the testicle and is most marked in the erect posture. It has been described frequently as "feeling like a bag of worms." Treatment consists of **excision of the varicose portion of the plexus**.

Torsion of the Testes

Twisting of the testes and terminal spermatic cord interferes with blood flow and leads to gangrene if not corrected within 4 hours of the onset of symptoms. There is a tendency toward bilaterality; therefore, bilateral orchidopexy should be performed at the time of detorsion. Torsion must commonly occurs in children and teenagers.

Phimosis and Paraphimosis

Phimosis is a condition in which the prepuce is elongated and the opening is so constricted that retraction cannot take place. Phimosis results in retention of secretions, with irritation and secondary infection. The treatment is **circumcision**.

Paraphimosis is a condition in which a tight, retracted prepuce is constricted behind the glans. There is swelling, edema, pain, and at times ulceration and gangrene. Most commonly, this occurs when the prepuce is not replaced after Foley catheterization. Early reduction of the paraphimosis may be performed by **manipulation**, but frequently it is necessary to make a **dorsal slit in the prepuce** to accomplish this. **Circumcision** should be performed unless infection is so extensive that the procedure must be deferred.

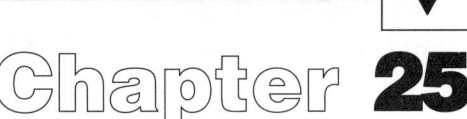

Chapter 25

Skin

The skin is an organ of astonishing complexity. It is a barrier between the relatively closed system of a human body and its external environment. It is strong, elastic, and waterproof; it is protective and self-repairing. In addition, it serves as a sense organ, an excretory organ, a heat control mechanism (involving the hair and sweat glands), and the organ of individual identification. This discussion includes some of the more common benign and malignant lesions of the skin.

BENIGN TUMORS

Seborrheic Keratosis

These common lesions occur everywhere on the body except on the palms of the hands and soles of the feet. They are dominantly inherited and appear after middle age. The lesions are raised and pigmented and often have verrucous surfaces that are friable and can easily be scraped off. **Cryotherapy** is the treatment of choice.

Keratoacanthoma

Clinically and histologically, this benign lesion **must be differentiated from squamous cell carcinoma**. It usually occurs in later years as a single lesion and is approximately 1 to 2 cm in diameter, with a characteristic horn-filled crater. The majority of solitary lesions arise from exposed areas. Keratoacanthomas are characterized by rapid growth, often reaching full size within a few weeks. Involution occurs spontaneously and is usually complete within 6 months. Treatment consists of first establishing the diagnosis. This is done by history and biopsy, which should include a section of adjoining normal skin.

Epidermal Cysts, Pilar Cysts, and Dermoid Cysts

These cysts are slow-growing, round, firm, intradermal or subcutaneous tumors that vary in size from 1 to 5 cm in diameter. The lesions frequently are solitary and commonly involve the face, scalp, neck, and trunk. Histologically, epidermoid cysts (incorrectly called sebaceous cysts) have a wall composed of true epidermis, and the cyst is filled with keratinaceous material. Treatment consists of **excision**. Pilar cysts are clinically indistinguishable from epidermoid cysts. Dermoid cysts usually are present at birth and are the result of sequestration of epidermal cells along lines of embryologic closure.

PREMALIGNANT TUMORS

Solar Keratosis

These lesions may be single or, more often, multiple. They appear on areas exposed to the sun in middle-aged, fair-complexioned persons. Prolonged exposure to the **sun** and **environmental carcinogens** are predisposing factors. Lesions are characterized by hyperkeratosis. It has been estimated that squamous cell carcinoma develops in 20% of patients. Lesions, both large and small, are treated with **cryotherapy** or topical **5-fluorouracil** (5-FU). Progress is favorable.

MALIGNANT TUMORS

Squamous Cell Carcinoma

Squamous cell carcinoma (SCC) can arise from the skin or from the oral or anal mucosa. Predisposing factors include exposure to the sun, chemical ingestion, chronic infection, chronic irritation, or irradiation. SCC arising from the oral mucosa, lips, anal mucosa, glans penis, vulva, and a long-standing sinus tract infection from osteomyelitis have a high rate of metastases. Treatment is dictated by location, predisposing factors, and degree of differentiation. Thus, a SCC arising from an area of solar keratosis can be **excised**. A more-aggressive approach is certainly indicated in SCC arising from a chronic focus of osteomyelitis, a chronic burn scar (Marjolin's ulcer), or previously irradiated areas.

Basal Cell Carcinoma

As indicated, basal cell carcinomas (BCC) are considered to be derivatives of pluripotential cells. They almost always occur in **areas of hair-bearing skin** and almost never in glabrous skin. Most BCC are undifferentiated. Treatment consists of **excision**. Metastases are rare.

Malignant Melanoma

Malignant melanoma (MM) is a neoplastic disorder produced by the malignant transformation of the normal melanocyte. **Melanocytes** are responsible for the production of melanin. During the first trimester of fetal life, precursor melanocytes arise from the **neural crest** and migrate to the skin, meninges, mucous membranes, upper esophagus, and eyes. In each of these locations, melanocytes have demonstrated the potential for malignant transformation. Currently, the risk of melanoma in the white population is 1 in 128.

Types of Melanoma

Melanoma is subdivided into four histopathologic types: (1) lentigo maligna melanoma, (2) superficial spreading, (3) acral lentiginous melanoma, and (4) nodular melanoma. The first three types have a junctional component, whereas **nodular melanoma is subjunctional**. Junctional melanomas proliferate in a horizontal direction initially, which is referred to as the radial growth phase. In time vertical growth appears, and this progression is associated with both invasive features and metastatic capabilities. **Subjunctional melanomas** usually demonstrate a predominant vertical growth phase and, therefore, have a very **early metastatic potential**.

Lentigo maligna melanoma is most commonly seen in individuals in their sixth to eighth decades of life. Superficial spreading melanoma occurs on areas of the body exposed to the sun and also those not exposed to the sun. It demonstrates a predominantly radial growth phase early.

Acral lentiginous melanoma is most commonly seen on the palms, soles, and subungual areas as well as on the mucous membranes. This also is the most common melanoma found in dark-pigmented people. It is associated with a poor clinical diagnosis.

In **multiple melanoma**, the extent of the malignancy at the time of diagnosis is the most important prognostic factor. The importance of **tumor thickness** predicting biologic behavior is noted by Breslow as follows: thickness of less than 0.76 mm is associated with local disease alone. More than 90% of these patients are cured with simple excision. Another schema for planning surgical management and any adjuvant regimen is using Clark's levels, as outlined in Table 25-1.

TABLE 25-1.
Clark's Levels of Tumor Invasion

Level	Description
1	All tumor cells above basement membrane
2	Invasion into loose connective tissue of papillary dermis
3	Tumor cells at junction of papillary reticular dermis
4	Invasion into reticular dermis
5	Invasion into subcutaneous fat

Treatment

A comprehensive treatment plan for melanoma is dependent on the accurate diagnosis and a complete assessment of histologic features that comprise the prognostic indicators. If the primary lesion is small, a **complete excisional biopsy** including the subcutaneous fat should be performed. If incisional biopsy is chosen, then the area of greatest tumor involvement should be selected. After diagnosis, **further wide-local excision** (>2-cm margin) should be undertaken. More complex lesions or those with lymph node involvement should undergo surgical evaluation, with flap coverage of the excised area and possible lymph node dissection.

Chapter 26

Vascular System

PERIPHERAL VASCULAR DISEASE

Atherosclerosis

Atherosclerosis is the most common cause of peripheral arterial occlusive disease. Patients with peripheral occlusive disease usually present with one or more of the following manifestations: asymptomatic, intermittent pain with exercise (claudication), persistent pain at rest, or tissue necrosis (with either ulceration or gangrene). **Asymptomatic patients** are those who are discovered to have arterial occlusive disease incidentally on physical examination, either with peripheral pulse deficits or the presence of an arterial bruit.

Claudication

Claudication is intermittent muscle pain caused by exercise and is relieved by a brief period of rest. It is important to differentiate true claudication from pseudoclaudication due to neurospinal or musculoskeletal conditions. Ischemic rest pain involves sharp or burning pain or numbness in the most distal aspect of the affected extremity, most commonly the toes and forefoot. Rest pain usually occurs at night and interferes with sleep. It is characteristically relieved by hanging the foot in a dependent position for a brief period or walking around the room.

Tissue Necrosis

Tissue necrosis represents the most severe expression of peripheral vascular disease. Ischemic ulceration usually occurs on the distal aspect of the extremity of the foot in areas predisposed to trauma, including the toes, dorsum of the foot, and malleoli. Ischemic ulcers are characterized by poor granulation tissue in the base and lack of epithelialization of the margins. Such ulcers should be differentiated from **venous stasis ulcers**, which usually occur on the medial aspect of the leg with a surrounding area of hyperpigmentation and stasis dermatitis. Venous stasis ulcers usually show good granulation tissue at the base and epithelialization at the margins when treated properly. **Gangrene** in peripheral vascular disease usually affects the toes, foot, and distal leg.

Surgical Management

Indications for surgery include four broad categories: (1) **life salvage**, such as repair of ruptured aortic aneurysm or arterial trauma or amputation for infected gangrene (Fig. 26-1); (2) **limb salvage**, with radiologic or surgical intervention to prevent limb loss secondary to gangrene, ischemic ulceration, or intolerable rest pain; (3) **preservation of function**, such as radiologic or surgical intervention to treat disabling claudication that limits self-care, occupation, or desired recreation; and (4) **prophylaxis**, such as repair of abdominal aortic aneurysm greater than 5 cm to prevent rupture, repair of popliteal aneurysm to prevent thrombosis and embolism, or carotid endarterectomy to prevent stroke. In the latter three conditions, an arteriogram is obtained preoperatively to assess vessels and plan surgical intervention.

Acute Arterial Occlusion

Acute arterial occlusion represents sudden obstruction of a peripheral artery by one of two principal mechanisms: **embolism or**

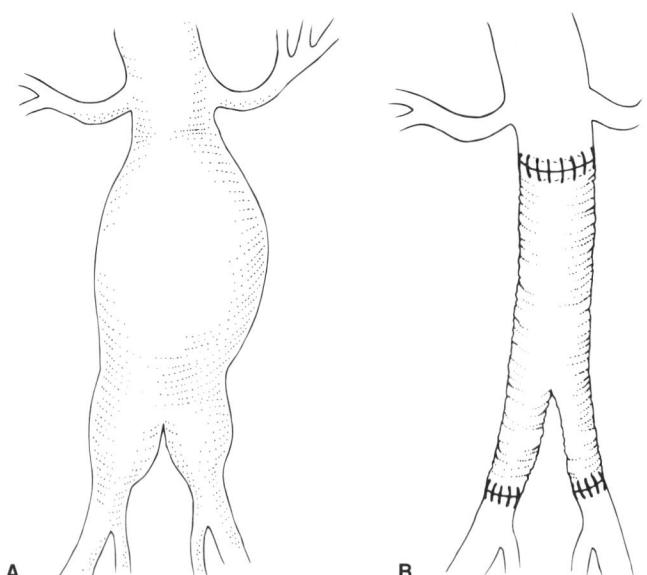

Figure 26-1.
A, Characteristic type of arteriosclerotic aneurysm arising below the renal arteries, involving both common iliac arteries.
B, Treatment by resection and replacement.

thrombosis. Acute arterial occlusion should be suspected in the presence of the five Ps, which include **pain, pallor, pulselessness, paresthesia,** and **paralysis.** Patients with acute arterial embolism should undergo Fogarty balloon catheter embolectomy. If arterial inflow is reestablished after a prolonged period of limb ischemia, **compartment syndrome** may develop. The anterior compartment in the leg is most commonly affected. A fasciotomy may be necessary to treat compartment syndrome.

DISORDERS OF THE VENOUS SYSTEM

Varicose Veins

Varicose veins of the lower extremity are an extremely common affliction, affecting **15% to 20% of the population**, with a female to male ratio of 5:1. They are classified as primary or secondary. **Primary** varicose veins are an isolated disorder of the superficial veins of the lower extremity and are not sequelae of deep venous thrombosis (DVT). **Secondary** varicosities are a manifestation of deep venous insufficiency and are associated with stigmata of chronic venous insufficiency, including edema, stasis dermatitis, skin pigmentation, ulceration, and the typical inflexible, scarred, woody appearance characteristic of the subcutaneous tissue. Details to suggest this condition should be carefully sought for during the history, because the pathophysiology and treatment are distinctly different from primary varicose veins. Minor involvement with primary varicose veins should be treated conservatively. Treatment options for more severe symptomatic (heavy sensation after prolonged standing) symptoms, which are refractory to conservative management, include excision or injection sclerotherapy.

Postphlebitic Syndrome

This syndrome is characterized by incompetence of the deep venous system. The syndrome arises most commonly as a consequence of **deep venous thrombosis (DVT)**. Postphlebitic syndrome may lead to secondary varicose veins. The treatment is conservative, with meticulous skin care, avoidance of local trauma, and the use of compression stockings. The patient should be advised of the chronic, relapsing, and **usually** incurable nature of this condition.

Pulmonary Embolism

Pulmonary embolism (PE) continues as a serious complication of a variety of primary medical and surgical disorders. The deep veins of the pelvis are the source of the emboli found in the pulmonary circulation. **Virchow's triad** characterizes the pathophysiology responsible for the formation of clots in the venous system and includes (1) stasis of the blood in the veins; (2) injury to the intimal surface of the veins, predisposing them to thrombosis; and (3) a generalized state of hypercoagulability. In addition, there are a number of predisposing factors in the development of **deep venous thrombosis** (DVT) including age, heart disease (particularly congestive heart failure [CHF] and atrial fibrillation), cancer, serious infections, and cerebrovascular accidents. Among the surgical procedures, DVT most commonly occurs after pelvic procedures (prostatectomy, hysterectomy), hip surgery, and knee procedures.

Diagnosis

The clinical manifestations of PE are dyspnea, chest pain, and hemoptysis. Clinical signs in order of incidence include tachycardia, fever, rales, tachypnea, and evidence of thrombophlebitis in the lower extremities. Asymptomatic PE is very common, because more than 50% of the pulmonary circulation must be occluded before serious physiologic changes are encountered. The chest radiograph may show evidence of diminished vascular marking in the area of pulmonary emboli (**Westermark's sign**). The electrocardiogram is seldom specific; however, arrhythmias and evidence of right heart strain may be seen.

Elevated alveolar-arterial PO$_2$ gradient is suggestive of PE. If the clinical symptomatology and baseline arterial blood gas results are suggestive of PE, a ventilation/perfusion (V/Q) scan should be done. Generally, this establishes the diagnosis. When the **ventilation/perfusion (V/Q) scan** shows intermediate probability for PE, a pulmonary angiogram should be obtained.

Treatment

After a firm diagnosis is made, the initial treatment consists of **anticoagulation therapy** with continuous administration of **heparin** and **bed rest** for 7 to 10 days to prevent further thrombosis. Administration of **warfarin** is begun several days before discontinuation of heparin and is maintained for 3 to 6 months. In those patients in whom heparin is contraindicated, an inferior vena cava filter can be placed radiologically through the femoral or internal jugular vein.

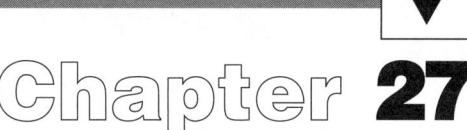

Chapter 27

Burns and Frostbite

Burns and injuries from cold constitute a major cause of morbidity and mortality. Attention to basic principles of initial trauma resuscitation and timely application of emergency measures minimize the morbidity and mortality of these injuries.

BURNS

The basic principles include high index of suspicion for the presence of airway compromise in smoke inhalation, the maintenance of hemodynamic stability, and fluid and electrolyte balance. After the airway is secure and the patient is given 100% oxygen, intravenous access (through burned skin if necessary) and administration of lactated Ringer's solution should be started. The volume of fluid is based on the area of burn: 4 mL/percent body surface area burned/kg mass; half the fluid should be administered over an 8-hour period beginning from time of injury, and the remaining half should be administered over a 16-hour period. This fluid is given in addition to maintenance intravenous fluids.

Extent and Depth of Burns

The **rule of nines** is a useful and practical guide to determine the extent of the burn. The **depth of the burn** is important in determining the severity of the injury. **First-degree** burns (e.g., sunburns) are characterized by erythema, pain, and the absence of blisters. **Second-degree**, or partial-thickness, burns are characterized by a red or mottled appearance with associated swelling and blister formation. The surface may have a weeping, wet appearance and is painful and hypersensitive, even to air current. Full-thickness, or **third-degree**, burns appear dark and leathery. The skin also may appear translucent and mottled or waxy white. The surface is painless and generally dry.

Treatment

For extensive burns, *cold compresses should not be applied* because hypothermia may result. Circulatory embarrassment in a circumferentially burned limb is best relieved by escharotomy. Fasciotomy is seldom required, but it may be necessary to restore circulation in patients with associated skeletal trauma, crush injury, high-voltage electrical injury, or burns involving the tissues beneath the investing fascia. Alkalization of the urine and maintenance of a urinary output of more than 100 mL/hour may be necessary in patients with electrical burns to prevent precipitation of myoglobin.

COLD INJURIES

Two types of cold injuries can be seen: (1) frostbite and (2) hypothermia. **Frostbite** is due to freezing of tissue from intracellular crystal formations and microvascular occlusion. Similar to thermal burns, frostbite is classified as first, second, third, and fourth degree, according to the depth of involvement. **First-degree** frostbite causes hyperemia and edema without skin necrosis. **Second-degree** frostbite manifests with vesicle formation accompanied by hyperemia and edema with partial-thickness skin necrosis. **Third-degree** frostbite is full-thickness necrosis with necrosis of some underlying subcutaneous tissue. **Fourth-degree** frostbite is full-thickness skin necrosis, including muscle and bone with gangrene.

Treatment

Treatment should be immediate rewarming, with the injured part placed in circulating water at 40°C until the pink color and perfusion returns. Dry heat should be avoided.

Hypothermia

Total-body hypothermia is defined as core temperature below 35°C. Clinically, hypothermia may be classified as **mild** (32° to 35°C), **moderate** (30°C to 32°C), or **severe** (below 30°C). The main **complication** of hypothermia is **cardiac arrhythmias**. Passive rewarming by elevation of room temperature and warm coverings is acceptable for the treatment of mild and moderate hypothermia. Severe hypothermia should be treated with active core-warming methods, including warmed peritoneal lavage or cardiopulmonary bypass.

Chapter 28

Fractures and Dislocations

A fracture is defined as a linear deformation or discontinuity of bone produced by forces that exceed the ultimate strength of the bone. Fractures are described anatomically according to location in the bone (intraarticular, epiphyseal, metaphyseal, diaphyseal), the plane of the fracture (transverse, oblique, spiral), the number and type of fragments, and whether the fracture is open (communication of the fracture with skin or mucous membrane) or closed. The clinical manifestations of fractures include pain, swelling, deformity, ecchymosis, instability, and crepitus. The diagnosis is usually confirmed radiologically, with two radiographs taken at right angles to each other. The injured extremity should always be examined carefully for neurovascular integrity.

OPEN FRACTURES

Open fractures represent a **surgical emergency**. In this situation, intravenous, empiric, broad-spectrum bacterial coverage should be given and the status of tetanus prophylaxis ascertained, followed by appropriate management. A puncture wound or communication of less than 1 cm in length defines a type I open fracture. Type II open fractures have a wound greater than 1 cm in length, with moderate associated soft tissue damage. Type III open fractures involve severe soft tissue injury and are divided into subtypes A (soft tissue injury only), B (severe soft tissue injury and bony injury/soft tissue loss), and C (associated neurovascular injury).

ASSOCIATED COMPLICATIONS

Compartment Syndrome

One of the most serious complications of extremity trauma or ischemic injury is compartment syndrome. The principal signs of diagnosis of this complication are **pain**, pallor, **paresthesias**, and ultimately **pulselessness**. This is in contradistinction to acute vascular insufficiency, in which pulselessness is an early manifestation. Tissue necrosis in compartment syndrome results from increased pressure and impairment of the flow in arterioles and capillaries. A reliable diagnosis of compartment syndrome is by measurement of the compartment pressures; pressures of 30 to 40 mm Hg constitute an indication for fasciotomy.

Fat Embolism Syndrome

Patients who sustain multiple fractures are at high risk for subsequent development of fat embolism, in which droplets of fat from the bone marrow enter the systemic circulation and impair pulmonary capillary perfusion by a complex mechanism. The final common pathway of fat embolism and other injuries that result from pulmonary parenchymal dysfunction following multisystem trauma is **adult respiratory distress syndrome (ARDS)**. Fat embolism generally occurs 24 to 72 hours after injury and presents with hypoxemia, tachycardia, tachypnea, fever, restlessness, and confusion. Petechiae may be present transiently, and **fat droplets are occasionally visible in blood specimens and urine**.

Ligamentous Injuries

Ligamentous injuries occur independent of bony injury and are referred to as sprains. Ligaments heal by progressive scar formation and contracture. Recent studies indicate that repair is improved by early motion in the absence of gross instability. Ligamentous injuries are graded as **type I** (stretch, but no disruption of fibers), **type II** (tear of some ligament fibers), and **type III** (complete mechanical discontinuity of the ligament). Types I and II generally are treated by immobilization or protected motion. Treatment of type III ligament injuries depends on many factors and can range from nonintervention (as for type III acromioclavicular separation) to immediate surgical repair or reconstruction (as indicated for a torn anterior cruciate ligament in a competitive athlete).

Traumatic Anterior Dislocation of the Shoulder

The cumulative range of motion of the shoulder is greater than any other joint. This is due to the lack of bony and soft tissue constraints. Acute traumatic **anterior dislocation is the most common** shoulder dislocation. It results from the forced abduction, extension, and external rotation of the shoulder. Following traumatic dislocation, the arm is held to the side, and the acromion process is prominent. The normal fullness of the shoulder is replaced by a concave contour just below the acromion. Evaluation must include a complete neurovascular examination because injury to the brachial plexus or axillary artery can occur. Radiographs confirm clinical diagnosis.

Reduction of the dislocation should be prompt. Reduction is accomplished by longitudinal traction on the arm with countertraction applied to the axilla. Once reduced, the arm is immobilized in a sling held in internal rotation for 3 weeks. Protected range of motion exercises are then initiated, but excessive abduction and external rotation should be avoided for 3 months. Recurrence is common in young patients and is less common in patients older than 40 years of age. In older patients, however, the rotator cuff frequently is torn at the time of dislocation.

Fractures of the Clavicle

The clavicle is an S-shaped bone that provides the only bony connection between the shoulder girdle and the axial skeleton. This is the first bone to ossify *in utero*. The clavicle is one of the most frequently fractured bones—especially in children. **Sixty percent** of all clavicle fractures **occur in children younger than 10 years of age**. Despite the proximity of the subclavian artery, pleura, and brachial plexus, injuries to these structures are uncommon. Most clavicular fractures require only **symptomatic treatment**. Support for the shoulder and arm can be provided with a stockinette bandage. A figure-of-eight bandage can assist in comfort.

Fractures of the Distal Forearm

Fractures of the distal radius and ulna are common in adults and children. The injury occurs by a fall on an outstretched arm with forces transmitted through the carpus, causing either volar or dorsal displacement. A **Colles' fracture** is a fracture of the distal radius with dorsal displacement and volar angulation (dinner fork deformity). Pain, swelling, and deformity are present just proximal to the wrist. Often a "step-off" in the distal radius can be appreciated by palpation. Median nerve function should always be tested because this nerve is susceptible to damage either by direct contusion or secondary compression. A Colles' fracture should be reduced under regional block by distraction.

Fractures of the Hip and Upper Femur

Fractures of the proximal femur occur most commonly in elderly women. Before the 20th century, fracture of the femur was almost universally fatal because of pulmonary, renal, and cardiac complications. Currently, the treatment of choice is **open and internal fixation**.

Fracture of the Carpal Scaphoid

The scaphoid bone is the **most commonly fractured carpal bone**. The scaphoid is the principal bony block to excessive dorsiflexion of the hand and wrist, and it is particularly susceptible to fracture during a fall on an outstretched hand. The most consistent sign of carpal injury is localized tenderness to digital pressure. Fracture of the carpal scaphoid produces tenderness to pressure in the anatomic "snuffbox," located between the extensor pollicis longus and the extensor pollicis brevis-abductor pollicis longus compartments.

The major problem that occurs when managing a scaphoid fracture is lack of early diagnosis and delay in initiation of treatment. If radiographs taken at the time of injury fail to show fracture but snuffbox tenderness persists, a cast should be applied and removed in 2 weeks, with repeat films completed. Bone resorption occurring by that time usually allows the fracture line to be visible. The major blood supply to the scaphoid is the radial artery. The majority of the branches enter through the dorsal surface, with blood flowing distal to proximal. The blood vessels are interrupted when the scaphoid fracture occurs, and the proximal segment becomes temporarily ischemic. **Missed diagnoses and late treatment** usually result in a **high incidence of nonunion and aseptic necrosis of the proximal fragment**. A properly applied cast is the treatment of choice.

DIRECTIONS: Each of the numbered items or incomplete statements in this section is followed by answers or by completions of the statement. Select the ONE lettered answer or completion that is BEST in each case.

1. A 56-year-old homeless man is found asleep on a curb. He is unresponsive. He is noted to have a core temperature of 27°C. The main complication of total body hypothermia with a temperature less than 30°C is

   (A) cardiac arrhythmias
   (B) hepatic insufficiency
   (C) impaired renal function
   (D) respiratory compromise

2. Which of the following statements regarding pancreatic cancer is correct?

   (A) Cancer of the exocrine pancreas most frequently occurs in the tail of the pancreas
   (B) Fewer than 10% of patients are surgically resectable at the time of diagnosis
   (C) Malignant endocrine tumors are more common than adenocarcinoma of the pancreas
   (D) Whipple's procedure is the appropriate operation for cancer of the tail of the pancreas

3. The mortality rate associated with septic shock is approximately

   (A) <10%
   (B) 20% to 30%
   (C) 50% to 70%
   (D) >90%

4. In which of the following situations does closed loop obstruction occur?

(A) When a loop of small bowel is twisted on an adhesion

(B) When the mesenteric vessels supplying a loop of bowel are occluded

(C) When there is a complete obstruction of the transverse colon in a patient with an incompetent ileocecal valve

(D) When there is a complete obstruction of the hepatic flexure in a patient with a competent ileocecal valve

5. Hyponatremia is asymptomatic until the sodium level falls below which amount?

(A) 135 mEq/L

(B) 130 mEq/L

(C) 125 mEq/L

(D) 120 mEq/L

6. A 55-year-old man presents with perineal pain, a "dragging" sensation along his inner thighs, and pain on defecation. The most appropriate initial management of this patient would consist of

(A) antibiotics

(B) prostatic massage

(C) Sitz baths

(D) transrectal drainage

7. In acute pancreatitis, mortality rates of 50% are found with which number of Ranson's criteria?

(A) 0 to 2

(B) 3 to 4

(C) 5 to 6

(D) >7

8. Two weeks after uncomplicated vaginal delivery, a 23-year-old woman presents with malaise, weakness, and a fluctuant, reddened area of her right breast. The most likely pathogen to be cultured is

(A) *Clostridia*

(B) Diphtheroids

(C) *Escherichia coli*

(D) *Staphylococcus aureus*

9. Of the following wounds described, which patient should receive tetanus immune globulin (TIG) and tetanus-diphtheria toxoid (Td) prophylaxis?

   (A) A 3-cm laceration on the forearm caused by a rusty blade; the patient is 23 years of age with a history of three Td immunizations
   (B) A 3-cm laceration on the forearm caused by a rusty blade; the patient is 23 years of age with a history of two Td immunizations
   (C) A 3-cm laceration on the forearm caused by a clean blade; the patient is 23 years of age with a history of three Td immunizations
   (D) A 3-cm laceration on the forearm caused by a clean blade; the patient is 23 years of age with a history of no Td immunizations

10. Which of the following conditions is followed by neurogenic shock?

    (A) Hemorrhage
    (B) High transection of the spinal cord
    (C) Sepsis
    (D) Toxemia

11. The incidence of lymph node metastases without a primary lesion is approximately

    (A) 1%
    (B) 4%
    (C) 8%
    (D) 10%

12. A 56-year-old diabetic patient presents with fever and chills. On history, he relates a pain in his anal region, with increased pain on defecation. On physical examination, a fluctuant tender, indurated area around his anus is noted. Appropriate initial management of this patient would be

    (A) intravenous antibiotics
    (B) oral antibiotics and steroid creams
    (C) prompt incision and drainage and antibiotic therapy
    (D) Sitz baths

13. Clinical features of neurogenic shock include which of the following terms?

   (A) Hypertension, bradycardia, and warm skin
   (B) Hypotension, bradycardia, and warm skin
   (C) Hypotension, tachycardia, and cool to clammy skin
   (D) Hypotension, tachycardia, and warm skin

14. Fractures of the carpal scaphoid are prone to nonunion and aseptic necrosis of the proximal fragment. This condition occurs

   (A) because blood flows from distal to proximal and fractures disrupt this flow
   (B) because intercarpal articular surfaces naturally pull the fracture apart
   (C) because tendinous insertion fractures naturally pull them apart
   (D) even though fractures are often detected early

15. Which of the following is the most common organism causing cellulitis?

   (A) *Haemophilus influenza*
   (B) *Streptococcus pneumoniae*
   (C) *Streptococcus pyogenes*
   (D) *Staphylococcus aureus*

16. Which of the following statements concerning snakebites is correct?

   (A) Antivenin should be given immediately to all patients with snakebites
   (B) The depth of the bite is generally one half of the distance between fang marks
   (C) There is a single antivenin available for all bites from pit vipers
   (D) Venom spread is largely via the blood stream

17. The maximum hourly administration of potassium to a patient with hypokalemia is

   (A) 10 mEq in 1 hour, with ECG monitoring
   (B) 20 mEq in 1 hour, with ECG monitoring
   (C) 40 mEq in 1 hour, with ECG monitoring
   (D) 60 mEq in 1 hour, with ECG monitoring

18. The principal mechanism of anticoagulant action of administering aspirin in low dosages is

    (A) induction of endothelial heparin production
    (B) induction of endothelial cell prostacyclin production
    (C) induction of capillary vasodilation
    (D) inhibition of platelet production of thromboxane A_2

19. A restrained patient has been brought to the emergency department with transverse linear ecchymosis on the abdominal wall. This physical finding should raise the concern of possible

    (A) intestinal injury
    (B) kidney injury
    (C) liver injury
    (D) splenic disruption

20. Erysipelas is a special type of cellulitis usually caused by which one of the following organisms?

    (A) *Escherichia coli*
    (B) *Haemophilus influenza*
    (C) *Staphylococcus aureus*
    (D) *Streptococcus pyogenes*

21. Which of the following groups of factors are vitamin K-dependent clotting factors?

    (A) Factors I, V, IX, and X
    (B) Factors II, VII, IX, and X
    (C) Factors I, VII, IX, and X
    (D) Factors II, VII, IX, and XI

22. Organ transplantations can occur without any medication between which of the following individuals?

    (A) Fraternal twins
    (B) Identical twins
    (C) Siblings
    (D) Cousins

23. A 41-year-old woman presents to your office and requests advice regarding mammography. Currently, mammography is recommended for which of the following groups?

    (A) Women ages 20 years and older under direction of a physician
    (B) Women ages 30 years and older under direction of a physician
    (C) Women between the ages of 40 and 50 years under direction of a physician
    (D) Recommended annually for women after the age of 40 years

24. A carbuncle is usually caused by

    (A) an infection of hair follicles
    (B) an insect bite
    (C) a severe sunburn
    (D) a subcutaneous injection of a medication

25. Which of the following statements concerning breast carcinoma *in situ* is correct?

    (A) Patients with surgically excised ductal carcinoma *in situ* (DCIS) are at low risk of developing invasive carcinoma of the ipsilateral breast
    (B) Lobular carcinoma *in situ* (LCIS) is part of a biologic continuum from atypical hyperplasia to invasive carcinoma
    (C) LCIS often progresses to invasive lobular carcinoma
    (D) LCIS usually is not a component of progressive disease that leads to invasive lobular carcinoma

26. Which of the following conditions is an example of vasogenic shock?

    (A) Acute myocardial infarction
    (B) Massive hemorrhage
    (C) Septic shock
    (D) Shock associated with multiple organ failure

Questions 27 and 28

27. A 3-year-old, otherwise healthy girl presents with a midline mass in her neck. This mass most likely originates from

    (A) the thyroid
    (B) the parathyroid
    (C) the pharyngeal floor at the base of the foramen cecum
    (D) the salivary glands

28. The most frequent location of the lesion described in this patient is

    (A) adjacent to the parathyroid glands
    (B) beneath the angle of the jaw
    (C) in the suprasternal notch
    (D) in the midline of the neck below the hyoid bone

29. Basic immunization with adsorbed tetanus toxoid requires which of the following treatment plans?

    (A) A single injection
    (B) One injection followed by a second in 4 to 6 weeks, and a third 6 to 12 months later
    (C) Three injections 2 weeks apart
    (D) One injection followed by annual injections for 2 years

30. Which of the following is the most appropriate treatment of hyperthyroidism in a young patient or a patient who is pregnant or lactating?

    (A) Iodides
    (B) Propylthiouracil
    (C) Radioactive iodine
    (D) Thyroid extract

31. Which of the following statements concerning the incidence and characteristics of gastric carcinoma is correct?

    (A) It commonly presents with symptoms suggestive of gastric ulcer
    (B) It is increasing in frequency in the United States
    (C) It occurs twice as often in females as in males
    (D) Ulcers due to gastric carcinoma and benign gastric ulcers are radiologically distinguishable

32. Which of the following statements concerning congenital heart lesions is correct?

   (A) 60% to 70% of atrial septal defects (ASD) frequently close before the age of 3 years
   (B) Patent foramen ovale is the same as an atrial septal defect (ASD)
   (C) The risk of endocarditis in ventricular septal defect (VSD) is small
   (D) Ventricular septal defects (VSD) are the most common congenital malformation of the heart

33. Which of the following statements concerning locoregional therapy for head and neck cancer is correct?

   (A) Definitive therapy refers to surgical resection of the tumor
   (B) For small tumors, surgical therapy provides a survival advantage compared with radiotherapy
   (C) Palliative procedures are justified even in the presence of distant disease
   (D) Radiotherapy is an effective method of managing large tumors (T2 or greater)

34. Which of the following definitions of shock is most accurate?

   (A) All patients with shock have associated hemorrhage
   (B) The primary basis of shock is bacteremia
   (C) Shock is a complication resulting primarily from toxins
   (D) Shock is a clinical syndrome caused by inadequate tissue perfusion

35. A newborn is noted on 1-week physical examination to be cyanotic. Arterial blood gas reveals a decreased PO_2. Which of the following could explain these findings?

   (A) Atrial septal defect (ASD)
   (B) Patent ductus arteriosus (PDA)
   (C) Tetralogy of Fallot
   (D) Ventricular septal defect (VSD)

36. Which of the following is usually the cause of tetanus?

   (A) Following a large abscess
   (B) Postoperative complication
   (C) Puncture wound
   (D) Superficial infection

37. A typical presenting sign of thyrotoxicosis is

   (A) atrial fibrillation
   (B) constipation
   (C) hair loss on the outer third of the eyebrows
   (D) low energy level

38. To obtain data concerning cardiac output, central venous pressure, and pulmonary wedge pressure, which of the following is the most appropriate procedure?

   (A) A catheter in the internal jugular vein
   (B) A catheter in the radial artery
   (C) A Swan-Ganz catheter in the pulmonary artery
   (D) A catheter in the right ventricular artery

39. Which of the following statements accurately describes primary varicose veins?

   (A) They affect 15% to 20% of the population
   (B) They cause venous stasis ulcers
   (C) They occur more frequently in men than in women
   (D) They predispose to the development of deep vein thrombosis

40. A patient is reported to have a potassium level of 7.3 mEq/L. The first diagnostic or therapeutic maneuver should include which of the following?

   (A) An ECG and infusion of glucose and insulin intravenously
   (B) An ECG and infusion of 45 mEq $NaHCO_3$
   (C) An ECG and administration of 1 g of 10% calcium gluconate
   (D) Transfer to an intensive care unit for careful cardiac monitoring

41. Which of the following characterizes the three phases of wound healing?

   (A) Epithelialization, contracture, and maturation
   (B) Inflammation, epithelialization, and contracture
   (C) Inflammation, fibroplasia, and maturation
   (D) Injury, fibroplasia, and maturation

42. A 63-year-old, otherwise healthy, man is undergoing inguinal hernia repair. When should prophylactic antibiotics be given to this patient?

(A) One single dose 1 hour before surgery
(B) 1 hour preceding surgery and for 24 hours following surgery
(C) For 24 hours preceding surgery and 24 hours after surgery
(D) For 48 hours preceding surgery and for 48 hours following surgery

43. The major risk for the administration of blood products is

(A) ABO incompatibility
(B) hemostatic breakdown
(C) hepatitis
(D) human immunodeficiency virus (HIV)

44. Following an automobile accident, a 33-year-old man is brought into the emergency department. He is tachycardiac (140 bpm), with cool and cyanotic extremities. His blood pressure is 90/36 mm Hg. Initial management of this patient should consist of which one of the following actions?

(A) Administration of ionotropic agents to increase cardiac output
(B) Administration of vasoconstrictors to increase peripheral vascular tone
(C) Administration of oxygen to increase the PO_2
(D) Infusion of crystalloids

45. Which of the following statements best describes melanocytes?

(A) They are derived from nerve cells in the epidermis
(B) They are found only in people with pigmented skin
(C) They arise from pluripotent cells in the basal layer of the skin
(D) They arise from the neural crest

46. In hemorrhagic pancreatitis, blood-stained fluid tracking along the falciform ligament to the umbilical region produces

(A) Caput Medusae
(B) Courvoisier's sign
(C) Cullen's sign
(D) Turner's sign

47. Warfarin impairs the formation of vitamin K-dependent factors by which of the following actions?

(A) Decreasing von Willebrand factor production
(B) Interfering with platelet production
(C) Reducing the amount of vitamin K available for gamma carboxylation
(D) Stimulating hepatic heparin production

48. An insensate burn appears dry, dark, and leathery and is known as a

(A) first-degree burn
(B) second-degree burn
(C) third-degree burn
(D) fourth-degree burn

49. The most common cause of a spontaneous pneumothorax is

(A) carcinoma of the lung
(B) pneumonia
(C) ruptured emphysematous bleb
(D) tuberculosis

50. Which of the following statements accurately describes chronic cholecystitis?

(A) It is characterized by intermittent, recurrent attacks of right upper quadrant pain usually following meals
(B) It is characterized by acute inflammation of the gallbladder usually associated with infection
(C) It implies the presence of gallstones in the common bile duct and can be associated with ascending cholangitis
(D) It denotes the presence of stones in the gallbladder but does not imply disease

51. Collagen accumulation in a wound is maximal by which of the following time periods?

(A) 10 days
(B) 21 days
(C) 42 days
(D) 6 months

52. Which of the following conditions is the most important aspect of total parenteral nutrition (TPN)?

(A) In those patients with high cholesterol, no lipids should be given
(B) It should be administered in a hospital setting with frequent blood sugar monitoring
(C) It should be administered at half levels when combined with enteral feeds
(D) Parameters and a goal for the TPN regimen should be established before the initiation of TPN

53. The osmolality of the serum is approximately

(A) 240 mOsm/L
(B) 270 mOsm/L
(C) 300 mOsm/L
(D) 330 mOsm/L

54. Which of the following adaptations in the metabolic response seen in chronic starvation is similar to that seen in the injured/stressed patient?

(A) Hepatic ketogenesis provides an alternate substrate for the central nervous system
(B) Metabolic rate is decreased
(C) Obligatory skeletal muscle breakdown occurs to support gluconeogenesis
(D) Oxygen consumption decreases

Questions 55 and 56

55. A 70-kg male patient has a measured serum sodium of 120 mEq/L (normal = 140 mEq/L). The calculated sodium deficit is

(A) 210 mEq
(B) 420 mEq
(C) 840 mEq
(D) 1050 mEq

56. To correct the serum sodium level of the above patient, the recommended maximum change of serum sodium in the first 24 hours would be

(A) 6 mEq/L in the first 24 hours
(B) 8 mEq/L in the first 24 hours
(C) 10 mEq/L in the first 24 hours
(D) 12 mEq/L in the first 24 hours

57. At what point is transfusion of red blood cells indicated?

(A) Hematocrit less than 25%
(B) Hematocrit less than 30%
(C) Blood loss of more than 500 mL blood without hemodynamic instability
(D) Blood loss of more than 500 mL blood with hemodynamic compromise

58. A postoperative patient is noted to have dyspnea and chest pain along with hemoptysis. Arterial blood gas, chest radiograph, and an electrocardiogram have been ordered. The next most appropriate investigation to document a pulmonary embolism would be

(A) chest fluoroscopy
(B) computed tomography (CT) scan
(C) pulmonary arteriogram
(D) ventilation/perfusion (V/Q) scan

59. Choledocholithiasis is most accurately described by which statement?

(A) It is characterized by intermittent, recurrent attacks of right upper quadrant pain usually following meals
(B) It is characterized by acute inflammation of the gallbladder usually associated with infection
(C) It denotes the presence of stones in the gallbladder but does not imply disease
(D) It implies the presence of gallstones in the common bile duct and can be associated with ascending cholangitis

60. The third-space fluid is a subcompartment of which of the following main compartments?

(A) Intracellular compartment
(B) Extracellular fluid compartment
(C) Intravascular fluid compartment
(D) Interstitial fluid compartment
(E) None of the above

61. The major histocompatibility complex (MHC) is located on which chromosome?

(A) Chromosome 4
(B) Chromosome 6
(C) Chromosome 12
(D) Chromosome 17

62. The amount of blood or fluid in the pericardial sac necessary to be removed to relieve the hemodynamic effects of acute pericardial tamponade is approximately

(A) 15 to 20 mL
(B) 50 mL
(C) 100 mL
(D) 150 mL

63. When compared with computed tomography (CT) in evaluation of abdominal trauma, a distinct disadvantage of diagnostic peritoneal lavage (DPL) is

(A) CT is faster
(B) DPL is more sensitive than the CT scan
(C) DPL is unsafe in unstable patients
(D) DPL is unable to assess the retroperitoneal structures

64. Overwhelming postsplenectomy sepsis is most commonly found in which age group?

(A) Children younger than 4 years of age and within 2 years after splenectomy
(B) Young females undergoing splenectomy for idiopathic thrombocytopenic purpura (ITP)
(C) Middle-aged patients undergoing splenectomy for trauma
(D) Elderly patients undergoing splenectomy for trauma

65. Which of the following is the best source of factor V?

  (A) Cryoprecipitate
  (B) Factor VIII concentrate
  (C) Fresh frozen plasma (FFP)
  (D) Prothrombin complex concentrate

66. Epidemiologically, fibroadenomas of the breast occur primarily in which of the following groups?

  (A) Girls younger than the age of 15 years
  (B) Women in their second and third decades
  (C) Women older than the age of 40 years
  (D) Occurs with approximately the same incidence in all age groups

67. In the United States, which of the following is the most common carcinoma of the thyroid?

  (A) Anaplastic
  (A) Follicular
  (C) Medullary
  (D) Papillary

68. Which of the following statements concerning pulmonary sequestration is correct?

  (A) It is often confused with diaphragmatic hernia
  (B) It receives its blood supply from a pulmonary vein, instead of the pulmonary artery
  (C) The sequestered lobe is prone to develop recurrent pulmonary infections
  (D) Ultrasound is the diagnostic study of choice

69. Most snakebite-related deaths in the United States follow a bite from which of the following snakes?

  (A) Copperhead
  (B) Cottonmouth
  (C) Rattlesnake
  (D) Water moccasin

70. Current indications for coronary artery bypass grafting include which of the following?

    (A) Those patients with a positive family history of coronary artery disease
    (B) Those patients with left main coronary artery disease
    (C) Those patients with coronary artery disease and renal failure
    (D) Those patients with medically well-controlled cardiac symptoms

71. The extracellular fluid represents approximately which percentage of total body water?

    (A) 5% to 15%
    (B) 15% to 25%
    (C) 25% to 35%
    (D) 35% to 45%
    (E) 45% to 55%

72. Which of the following statements concerning gynecomastia is correct?

    (A) It can be induced by anabolic steroids
    (B) Gynecomastia predisposes to male breast cancer
    (C) Physiologic gynecomastia occurs during two phases of life
    (D) Total mastectomy is a treatment of choice in managing the disease

73. Overadministration of diuretics is associated with which one of the following conditions?

    (A) Anion gap metabolic acidosis
    (B) Chloride-responsive metabolic alkalosis
    (C) Chloride-unresponsive metabolic alkalosis
    (D) Nonanion gap metabolic acidosis

74. A patient returns from a vacation in South America where she was bitten by a dog. Which of the following is the best treatment of suspected rabies?

    (A) Manage by local wound care and systemic antibiotics
    (B) Treat with vaccine prophylaxis in appropriate cases
    (C) Treat by wide, total excision of the injured site
    (D) Wait for information about the dog from South American contacts

75. Of the following figures, what is the approximate normal daily secretion from the salivary glands?

    (A) 250 mL
    (B) 500 mL
    (C) 750 mL
    (D) >1000 mL

76. The major differential diagnosis for keratoacanthoma is

    (A) basal cell carcinoma
    (B) melanoma
    (C) solar keratosis
    (D) squamous cell carcinoma

77. Which of the following conditions may result if hypernatremia is corrected too rapidly?

    (A) Central pontine myelinolysis
    (B) Convulsions and coma
    (C) Hyperkalemia
    (D) Oliguric renal failure

78. The most effective way to control wound contracture is

    (A) administration of vitamin E systemically
    (B) application of corticosteroid cream to wound
    (C) full-thickness skin graft to wound
    (D) split-thickness skin graft to wound

79. Addition of isotonic saline to the intravascular space results in

    (A) increase in intracellular fluid volume and increase in extracellular fluid volume
    (B) increase in only intracellular volume
    (C) increase in only extracellular volume
    (D) increase in extracellular fluid and a decrease in intracellular volume

80. Which of the following statements accurately describes fat embolism syndrome?

    (A) It is seen within 12 hours after a patient has sustained multiple fractures
    (B) Fat droplets occasionally are visible in the blood and urine
    (C) It rarely has any significant sequelae
    (D) It results from fat from adipose cells entering the blood stream

81. Which of the following is the best source of fibrinogen?

    (A) Cryoprecipitate
    (B) Factor VIII concentrate
    (C) Fresh frozen plasma (FFP)
    (D) Prothrombin complex concentrate

82. Which of the following cells are essential to wound healing?

    (A) Basophils
    (B) Eosinophils
    (C) Macrophages
    (D) Neutrophils

83. What percentage of patients with head and neck cancer die because of locoregional disease?

    (A) 20%
    (B) 30%
    (C) 40%
    (D) 50%
    (E) 60%

84. Postoperative chemoradiation therapy for colon cancer is recommended for the patient with which stage of cancer?

    (A) Dukes' A
    (B) Dukes' B
    (C) Dukes' C
    (D) Dukes' D

85. Which of the following best describes pseudocysts?

    (A) They are always associated with pancreatitis
    (B) They always represent benign pathophysiology
    (C) They should be left alone if more than 5 cm in diameter
    (D) They are characterized by a lack of a true epithelial cell lining

86. The majority of salivary gland tumors are located in which of the following glands?

    (A) Mucous glands of the hard and soft palate
    (B) Parotid glands
    (C) Sublingual glands
    (D) Submaxillary glands

87. The role of the polymorphonuclear lymphocyte in wound healing is to

    (A) phagocytize bacteria
    (B) produce antibodies
    (C) raise local temperature
    (D) secrete antibiotic substances

88. Which of the following most correctly describes a felon?

    (A) A closed space infection of the distal phalanx
    (B) An infection of the extensor tendon of the hand
    (C) An infection of the palmar space
    (D) A subungual infection

89. Which of the following statements best describes mammography?

    (A) It is an effective screening study for breast cancer
    (B) It is a screening study that should be obtained by women at age 50 years
    (C) It should not be used as a substitute for a biopsy
    (D) It is not indicated in the presence of a palpable breast mass

90. The parotid gland drains into the mouth via which of the following ducts?

    (A) Stensen's duct
    (B) The duct of Santorini
    (C) The ducts of Luschka
    (D) Wharton's duct

91. In the United States, cancer of the breast statistically is

    (A) the leading cause of cancer-related deaths
    (B) the second leading cause of cancer-related deaths
    (C) the third leading cause of cancer-related deaths
    (D) the fourth leading cause of cancer-related deaths

92. Riedel's thyroiditis is associated with which of the following conditions?

    (A) A bacterial infection
    (B) A neoplastic disorder
    (C) Invasive fibrous thyroiditis
    (D) Tuberculosis

93. Transillumination of the scrotum may help distinguish which of the following conditions?

    (A) A hydrocele
    (B) Testicular cancer
    (C) Torsion of the testicle
    (D) A varicocele

94. A 35-year-old woman presents with a palpable mass. The quickest, most cost-effective approach to establish the diagnosis of breast cancer in this patient would be

    (A) excisional biopsy
    (B) fine-needle aspiration (FNA)
    (C) mammography
    (D) stereotactically guided biopsy

95. Which one of the following melanomas is associated with early metastases?

    (A) Acral lentiginous melanoma
    (B) Lentigo maligna melanoma
    (C) Nodular melanoma
    (D) Superficial spreading melanoma

96. Which of the following descriptions best characterizes Paget's disease of the breast?

    (A) It is a chronic eczematous eruption of the nipple
    (B) It is an allergic disorder
    (C) It frequently follows irradiation of the breast
    (D) It usually is a benign and self-limited disorder

97. The operation for duodenal ulcer with the lowest risk of recurrence is

    (A) highly selective vagotomy
    (B) Nissen fundoplication
    (C) vagotomy and antrectomy
    (D) vagotomy and pyloroplasty

98. Which of the following statements concerning carcinoma of the breast is correct?

    (A) It occurs in one of eight women in the United States
    (B) It usually presents with bloody nipple discharge
    (C) Patients usually present with a painful breast mass
    (D) Women frequently have clinically detectable metastatic disease at the time of the initial diagnosis

99. In flail chest, the hypoxemia stems from which of the following conditions?

    (A) Associated hemothorax
    (B) Damage to the underlying lung parenchyma
    (C) Paradoxical movement of the segment of ribs
    (D) Poor respiration secondary to pain from multiple broken ribs

100. Which of the following statements concerning fibroadenomas of the breast is correct?

    (A) They display no estrogen sensitivity
    (B) They often are fixed to the underlying pectoral fascia
    (C) They should all be removed because of the malignant potential
    (D) They sometimes present with concurrent lobular carcinoma *in situ*

101. Hashimoto's disease of the thyroid is thought to be primarily

    (A) an autoimmune disorder
    (B) fibrotic obliteration of the gland
    (C) neoplastic
    (D) tuberculous in origin

102. Which of the following is a characteristic of lung abscesses?

    (A) They are most commonly caused by aspiration
    (B) They are treated with lung resection
    (C) They are indistinguishable radiographically from pneumonia
    (D) They rarely require antibiotic therapy if they are well drained

103. Which of the following statements accurately describes nephrolithiasis?

    (A) 90% of renal calculi are radiolucent
    (B) 1% to 3% of the adult population is affected by nephrolithiasis
    (C) Surgical removal is required for the majority of patients with nephrolithiasis
    (D) Urinalysis does not show any red blood cells in 50% of patients with nephrolithiasis

104. Which of the following statements most accurately describes benign prostatic hypertrophy (BPH)?

   (A) By age 80 years, 50% of men have evidence of BPH
   (B) It is a precursor to prostatic cancer
   (C) It can have significant impact on the quality of life
   (D) It is second to cancer as the most common disease of the prostate

105. Which of the following thyroid neoplasms produce calcitonin?

   (A) Anaplastic
   (B) Follicular
   (C) Medullary
   (D) Papillary

106. Which of the following statements concerning fine-needle aspiration (FNA) for breast masses is correct?

   (A) A negative nondiagnostic FNA should be followed by repeat mammography in 12 months
   (B) False-positives are frequent
   (C) It can be used for nonpalpable masses detected by mammography
   (D) The false-negative interpretation varies from center to center but is generally 30%

107. Generally, wound infection rates for clean wounds are *less than* what percentage?

   (A) 1%
   (B) 3%
   (C) 5%
   (D) 10%

108. A patient presents complaining of "heartburn." The most accurate way to diagnose gastroesophageal reflux disease (GERD) is

   (A) demonstration of a hypotensive lower esophageal sphincter
   (B) documentation of a hiatal hernia
   (C) history of heartburn
   (D) measuring the number of hours the pH is less than 4

109. Of the following ratios, which indicates the approximate current risk of melanoma in the white population?

    (A) 1 in 50
    (B) 1 in 150
    (C) 1 in 500
    (D) 1 in 1000

110. In the Unites States, the most common cause of acute pancreatitis is

    (A) alcohol
    (B) drug allergy
    (C) gallstones
    (D) hyperlipidemia

111. The rate of infection for a contaminated wound is

    (A) 2% to 3%
    (B) 3% to 5%
    (C) 8% to 10%
    (D) 15% to 30%

112. Which of the following shoulder dislocations is most common?

    (A) Anterior
    (B) Inferior
    (C) Lateral
    (D) Posterior

113. Which of the following is the best treatment option for patients with lobular carcinoma *in situ* (LCIS)?

    (A) Bilateral radical mastectomy
    (B) Hormonal treatment
    (C) Lifelong observation of both breasts with mammography and physical examination
    (D) Wide local excision of the affected area, followed by external beam radiotherapy

114. Which of the following is the only contraindication to diagnostic peritoneal lavage (DPL) or computed tomography (CT)?

    (A) The patient has a pressing need for exploratory laparotomy
    (B) The patient is obtunded from ethanol ingestion
    (C) The patient is obtunded from severe head trauma
    (D) The patient is pregnant

115. Which of the following accurately describes cholelithiasis?

    (A) It is characterized by intermittent, recurrent attacks of right upper quadrant pain, usually following meals
    (B) It is characterized by acute inflammation of the gallbladder, usually associated with infection
    (C) It denotes the presence of stones in the gallbladder but does not imply disease
    (D) It implies the presence of gallstones in the common bile duct and can be associated with ascending cholangitis

116. A patient presents with a pigmented nevus. You perform an excisional biopsy and send it to the laboratory for microscopic analysis. You would expect an almost 90% cure rate with simple excision alone if the Breslow level was

    (A) <0.16 mm
    (B) <0.46 mm
    (C) <0.76 mm
    (D) <1.56 mm

117. The pathophysiology of appendicitis is

    (A) a closed loop obstruction
    (B) edema of the appendix
    (C) infarction to the appendix
    (D) ulceration of the appendiceal mucosa

118. A 59-year-old woman presents to your office with a chest radiograph demonstrating an anterior mediastinal mass. The most common anterior mediastinal mass is

    (A) lymphoma
    (B) neurilemoma
    (C) pericardial cyst
    (D) thymoma

119. The predominant clinical feature of acute pancreatitis is

    (A) crampy abdominal pain associated with nausea and vomiting
    (B) dull, periumbilical pain
    (C) penetrating epigastric pain, radiating to the back
    (D) sudden, stabbing epigastric pain

120. Which of the following statements most accurately describes treatment of hip fractures?

    (A) They are best treated with open reduction and internal fixation

    (B) They can be treated with bed rest and traction with good results

    (C) They should be treated with a lower body cast

    (D) They are best treated with total hip replacement

121. A 35-year-old woman presents with a groin mass. Which of the following is the most common cause of this mass?

    (A) Epigastric hernia

    (B) Femoral hernia

    (C) Inguinal hernia

    (D) Umbilical hernia

122. The most common cause of chronic pancreatitis in the United States is

    (A) alcohol

    (B) drug allergy

    (C) gallstones

    (D) hyperlipidemia

123. Esophageal varices result from portosystemic anastomoses between which of the following veins?

    (A) The left gastric vein

    (B) The retroperitoneal veins

    (C) The short gastric and gastroepiploic veins

    (D) The umbilical and periumbilical veins

124. Which of the following statements accurately describes right-sided colon cancers?

    (A) They are infrequently associated with anemia

    (B) They are often small lesions

    (C) They frequently have metastatic disease at the time of presentation

    (D) They usually present as obstructing lesions

125. Which feature most accurately distinguishes Crohn's disease from ulcerative colitis (UC)?

(A) Ileum is devoid of disease in ulcerative colitis
(B) Increased incidence of cancer in Crohn's disease only
(C) Toxic megacolon is found only in Crohn's disease
(D) Transmural disease noted on microscopic analysis in Crohn's disease

126. Which of the following statements correctly describes acute cholecystitis?

(A) It is characterized by intermittent, recurrent attacks of right upper quadrant pain usually following meals
(B) It is characterized by acute inflammation of the gallbladder usually associated with infection
(C) It denotes the presence of stones in the gallbladder but does not imply disease
(C) It implies the presence of gallstones in the common bile duct and can be associated with ascending cholangitis

127. A 5-year-old patient who sustains a minor wound with a clean razor blade comes to the emergency department. His previous tetanus immunization status is unknown. In the emergency room, his wound should be cleaned and sutured. Which of the following is the next step in treating this patient?

(A) The patient should receive Td (tetanus-diphtheria toxoid)
(B) The patient should receive DPT (diphtheria-pertussis-tetanus)
(C) The patient should receive Td (tetanus-diphtheria) and TIG (tetanus immune globulin)
(D) The patient should *not* receive any tetanus prophylaxis because the wound is a minor wound and it is clean

128. Which one of the following features about clavicular fractures is correct?

(A) They are most common in the elderly
(B) They frequently cause injury to surrounding structures
(C) They are prone to nonunion
(D) Most require only symptomatic treatment

129. Overwhelming postsplenectomy infection is associated in more than 50% of cases with which organism?

(A) *Haemophilus influenzae*
(B) Parvovirus
(C) *Staphylococcus aureus*
(D) *Streptococcus pneumoniae*

130. A 55-year-old woman, who had a hysterectomy 10 years previously, presents with a partial small bowel obstruction. You elect to start her on intravenous fluids and nasogastric suction. In such patients with partial small bowel obstruction, the percentage who eventually require operative intervention is

(A) 10%
(B) 20%
(C) 30%
(D) 40%

131. A 15-year-old boy falls off his bicycle and breaks his humerus. Following reduction of a closed fracture, important steps in management of this patient would include all of the following EXCEPT

(A) checking for neurovascular integrity of the involved extremity
(B) immobilizing the extremity
(C) obtaining radiographs of the extremity
(D) starting intravenous antibiotics

132. All of the following statistics about pheochromocytoma are true EXCEPT

(A) 10% are benign
(B) 10% are bilateral
(C) 10% are extraadrenal

133. Which of the following is NOT an example of a clean-contaminated wound?

(A) Cholecystectomy for chronic cholecystitis
(B) Common bile duct exploration for ascending cholangitis
(C) Nephrectomy for hydronephrosis
(D) Pulmonary resection for a pulmonary nodule

134. All of the following statements regarding carcinoid tumor of the small bowel are correct EXCEPT

   (A) it metastasizes more than carcinoid tumors anywhere else in the intestinal tract
   (B) it can produce carcinoid syndrome without metastases to the liver
   (C) carcinoid syndrome is caused by excessive levels of serotonin
   (D) diagnosis of carcinoid is confirmed by finding increased levels of urinary 5-hydroxyindoleacetic acid (5-HIAA)

135. All of the following statements concerning total body water are true EXCEPT

   (A) total body water constitutes 50% to 70% of total body weight
   (B) total body water increases with age
   (C) increasing body fat causes a decrease in total body water
   (D) total body water is less in a female compared with a male of the same weight

136. Which of the following statements concerning head and neck cancers is NOT true?

   (A) Incidence is higher in males than in females
   (B) Incidence and mortality rates have remained relatively stable in nonwhite males and females
   (C) Late-stage presentation is uncommon
   (D) Symptoms referable to the tumor itself are mild and do not necessarily correlate with the size of the tumor

137. A man presents to the emergency department after an automobile crash. He is in respiratory distress. Which of the following conditions would NOT suggest the diagnosis of right-sided tension pneumothorax?

   (A) Decreased breath sounds on the right
   (B) Distention of the neck veins
   (C) Distant heart sounds
   (D) Tracheal deviation to the left

138. Which of the following statements concerning surgical drains is NOT true?

   (A) Drains should be omitted in clean cases where soilage is minimal
   (B) Drains should be placed routinely after intraabdominal surgery so that the peritoneal cavity is well drained
   (C) Except for chest tubes, drains are generally poor indicators of postoperative bleeding
   (D) Penrose drains are considered open drains

139. All of the following statements concerning compartment syndrome are true EXCEPT

   (A) it is seen following extremity trauma or ischemia
   (B) pain is an early symptom
   (C) pressures of 30 to 40 mm Hg constitute an indication for fasciotomy
   (D) pulselessness is an early clinical manifestation

140. A 67-year-old man presents with dysphagia. All of the following are suggestive of esophageal cancer in this patient EXCEPT

   (A) history of smoking
   (B) history of columnar metaplasia
   (C) midsternal chest pain
   (D) weight loss of 35 lb in the past year

141. Which clinical sign is NOT associated with cardiac tamponade?

   (A) Beck's triad
   (B) Kussmaul's sign
   (C) Murphy's sign
   (D) Pulsus paradoxus

142. An increase in which of the following enzyme levels does NOT imply cholestasis?

   (A) Alanine aminotransferase (ALT)
   (B) Alkaline phosphatase
   (C) Gamma glutamyltransferase (GGT)
   (D) 5'-nucleotidase (5'-N)

143. Substances secreted in saliva include all of the following EXCEPT

    (A) albumin
    (B) amylase
    (C) immunoglobulins A, G, and M
    (D) lysozyme
    (E) trypsin

144. Which of the following statements concerning nutrition in the surgical patient is NOT true?

    (A) A minimum of 100 g of glucose daily is required to minimize the protein catabolism
    (B) Gastrostomy feeds are generally acceptable in any patient who is not ventilated
    (C) The preferred method of feeding a patient with a functional gastrointestinal tract is by enteral feeds
    (D) The majority of surgical patients do not require a special nutritional regimen

145. All of the following are appropriate in the management of cellulitis EXCEPT

    (A) antibiotics
    (B) application of heat
    (C) elevation of the affected extremity
    (D) incision and drainage

146. Parathyroid hormone (PTH) level is increased in all of the following conditions EXCEPT

    (A) hypercalcemia due to metastases
    (B) primary hyperparathyroidism
    (C) secondary hyperparathyroidism
    (D) tertiary hyperparathyroidism

147. Which of the following would NOT increase the suspicion of thyroid malignancy in a solitary thyroid nodule?

    (A) A history of previous radiation exposure to the head and neck
    (B) Age older than 40 years in men and older than 50 years in women
    (C) A hypofunctional nodule by scintillation scan
    (D) Female gender

148. Which information is NOT necessary before surgical intervention for gastroesophageal reflux disease (GERD) is attempted?

(A) Demonstration of a defective lower esophageal sphincter mechanism
(B) Esophagitis by endoscopy
(C) Increased esophageal exposure to gastric juice on a 24-hour pH study
(D) Presence of adequate esophageal contractions

149. All of the following agents are commonly isolated in the bile of patients with acute cholecystitis EXCEPT

(A) *Bacteroides fragilis*
(B) *Enterococcus*
(C) *Escherichia coli*
(D) *Klebsiella*

150. All of the following statements concerning sutures are true EXCEPT

(A) in the face of infections, nonabsorbable sutures act as foreign bodies and perpetuate infection
(B) metal sutures are devoid of tissue reaction
(C) monofilament sutures are less conducive to infection than multifilament sutures of the same material
(D) silk is the only suture currently used that is not synthetic

151. Which of the following statements concerning rabies is NOT true?

(A) A patient who has had contact with the blood, urine, or feces of a rabid animal should undergo rabies prophylaxis
(B) An unprovoked attack by a domestic animal is a common scenario leading to rabies exposure
(C) Bites on the hand and face carry the highest risk of causing rabies
(D) Exposure to a dog outside of the United States is the most common cause of rabies in the Unites States

152. All of the following are major causes of small bowel obstruction EXCEPT

    (A) adhesions
    (B) gallstone ileus
    (C) hernias
    (D) malignant tumors

153. Which of the following statements concerning hemostasis is NOT correct?

    (A) Factor VII has the shortest half-life
    (B) Heparin inhibits coagulation by forming a complex with antithrombin III
    (C) The effect of warfarin can be counteracted by administration of vitamin K
    (D) The effect of heparin can be reversed by transfusion with fresh frozen plasma (FFP)

154. Which of the following statements concerning breast cysts is NOT true?

    (A) Cysts rarely require excision, except if the aspirate is bloody
    (B) Patients with fibrocystic disease often present with diffuse breast pain, often accentuated during the second half of the menstrual cycle
    (C) Single dominant cysts should be aspirated
    (D) There is an increased risk of breast cancer in patients with fibrocystic breast disease

155. In a patient with increased anion gap metabolic acidosis, all of the following clinical situations can be found EXCEPT

    (A) diabetic ketoacidosis
    (B) ethylene glycol ingestion
    (C) hypovolemic shock
    (D) pancreatic fistula
    (E) renal failure

156. A patient undergoes a partial gastrectomy for ulcer disease. In his preoperative counseling, you mention the dumping syndrome to him. All of the following characterize dumping syndrome EXCEPT

(A) it occurs after partial gastric resections
(B) patients often experience faintness, sweating, palpitations, and nausea after ingestion of food
(C) patients often experience vomiting
(D) treatment is aimed at increasing fat intake, decreasing carbohydrate intake, and restricting liquids to between meals

157. All of the following are indications for surgical intervention in a patient with peripheral vascular disease EXCEPT

(A) acute arterial occlusion
(B) new onset claudication
(C) rest pain
(D) tissue necrosis

158. In a patient who is involved in an automobile accident, which of the following would NOT preclude the placement of a urinary bladder catheter?

(A) A high-riding prostate noted on physical examination
(B) A history of prostatic hypertrophy
(C) An ecchymotic scrotum
(D) Blood in the urethral meatus

159. Which of the following statements concerning the rabies vaccines is NOT true?

(A) Human rabies immune globulin (HRIG) is given only if the risk of exposure is high
(B) Human rabies immune globulin (HRIG) and human diploid cell vaccine (HDCV) should *not* be given together
(C) Injection of either rabies vaccine should *not* be administered in the gluteal region, because it results in a reduction in the neutralizing antibody titers
(D) There are currently two vaccines available: human diploid cell vaccine (HDCV) and rabies vaccine adsorbed (RVA)

160. All of the following retard wound healing EXCEPT

   (A) decreased PO_2
   (B) deficiency of vitamin C
   (C) low blood flow
   (D) hypoglycemia

161. All of the following are complications of diverticular disease of the colon EXCEPT

   (A) bleeding
   (B) obstruction
   (C) perforation
   (D) perianal fistula

162. Of the following organs, which has NOT been successfully transplanted clinically?

   (A) Left lobe of the liver
   (B) Pancreatic islet cells
   (C) Right lung
   (D) Spinal cord

163. Which of the following statements regarding lung cancer is NOT true?

   (A) Bronchogenic carcinoma is seen predominantly in men between the ages of 55 and 60 years
   (B) Cough is the principal presenting symptom
   (C) Lung cancer is the most common cause of cancer-related deaths in both women and men
   (D) Small cell lung cancer (SCLC) has a relatively good prognosis compared with non-small cell lung cancer (NSCLC)

164. Of the four major classes of carcinoma of the thyroid, which is the LEAST invasive?

   (A) Anaplastic
   (B) Follicular
   (C) Medullary
   (D) Papillary

165. Thyrotoxicosis is associated with all of the following conditions EXCEPT

   (A) Graves' disease
   (B) Riedel's thyroiditis
   (C) toxic adenoma
   (D) toxic multinodular goiter

166. Parathyroid hormone has an effect on all of the following EXCEPT it

    (A) enhances intestinal absorption of calcium and phosphates
    (B) increases resorption of calcium in the kidney
    (C) responds to an increase in serum calcium by decreasing secretion
    (D) stimulates calcium resorption in the bone

167. Virchow's triad, which characterizes the pathophysiology associated with deep venous thrombosis (DVT), includes all of the following EXCEPT

    (A) hypercoagulability
    (B) intimal injury
    (C) stasis
    (D) varicose veins

168. Which of the following conditions is NOT associated with multiple endocrine neoplasia type I (MEN-I)?

    (A) Hyperparathyroidism
    (B) Medullary carcinoma of the thyroid
    (C) Pancreatic neoplasm
    (D) Pituitary neoplasm

169. A 57-year-old man with a long history of tobacco abuse presents to your office with a chest radiograph demonstrating a single 4-cm lesion in the right upper lobe. To ascertain the resectability of the lesion, you would order all of the following tests EXCEPT

    (A) Bone scan
    (B) Bronchoscopy
    (C) Computed tomography (CT) of the chest
    (D) Pulmonary function tests

170. Surgical therapy for peptic ulcer disease (PUD) has decreased with the advent of pharmacologic agents that control and decrease gastric acid secretion. However, surgery is still necessary under several conditions. All of the following are indications for surgical intervention in the management of peptic ulcer disease EXCEPT

    (A) gastric outlet obstruction
    (B) intractable bleeding
    (C) night pain
    (D) perforation of an ulcer

171. Increasingly, breast-conservation therapy is being used in the management of invasive carcinoma. A patient presents to your clinic and requests breast conservation. You would mention to her that all of the following are contraindications to breast conservation therapy EXCEPT

(A) collagen vascular disease
(B) lack of patient commitment to undergo irradiation and/or close follow-up
(C) lobular carcinoma *in situ* (LCIS)
(D) multifocal primary tumors

172. All of the following are major characteristics of the liver EXCEPT

(A) center for acid-base control
(B) dual blood supply
(C) enterohepatic circulation
(D) regenerative capacity

173. Which of the following statements concerning tumors of the salivary glands is NOT true?

(A) 80% of parotid tumors are benign
(B) 80% of the benign parotid tumors are pleomorphic adenomas
(C) Pleomorphic adenomas occur most frequently in the fifth decade with a slight male predominance
(D) Tumors can arise from any of the mucous glands of the hard and soft palate

174. All of the following suggest airway injury in a burned patient EXCEPT

(A) a burned face
(B) carbonaceous sputum
(C) a burned upper chest
(D) singed nasal hair

175. Which of the following is NOT an absorbable suture?

(A) Dexon
(B) Plain cat gut
(C) Silk
(D) Vicryl

176. Which of the following is NOT a normal area of esophageal narrowing?

    (A) The diaphragmatic hiatus
    (B) The entrance to the esophagus
    (C) The indentation due to the left main-stem bronchus and the aortic arch
    (D) The indentation due to the right atrium

177. Zollinger-Ellison syndrome is characterized by all of the following EXCEPT

    (A) patient frequently presents with ulcers and constipation
    (B) patient will have gastric acid hypersecretion
    (C) patient will have increased serum gastrin levels
    (D) patient will have a paradoxical increase in serum gastrin in response to intravenous secretion

178. All of the following are features of tetralogy of Fallot EXCEPT

    (A) dextroposition of the aorta
    (B) hypertrophy of the left ventricle
    (C) obstruction of the right ventricular outflow tract
    (D) ventricular septal defect

179. Which of the following conditions is NOT characteristic of cardiogenic shock?

    (A) Arrhythmia
    (B) Decreased cardiac output
    (C) Massive blood loss
    (D) Myocardial infarction

180. Which of the following is NOT a cardinal sign or symptom of intestinal obstruction?

    (A) Abdominal distention
    (B) Diarrhea
    (C) Episodic abdominal pain
    (D) Obstipation
    (E) Vomiting

181. The classic triad in renal cell carcinoma includes all of the following signs and symptoms EXCEPT

   (A) abdominal mass
   (B) flank pain
   (C) hematuria
   (D) lower body swelling from vena caval obstruction

182. Which of the following conditions has NOT been shown to alter wound healing in a sterile wound?

   (A) Diabetes mellitus
   (B) Malignancy
   (C) Neutropenia
   (D) Renal insufficiency

DIRECTIONS: Each set of matching questions in this section consists of a list of three to twenty-six options followed by several numbered items. For each numbered item, select the ONE lettered option that is most closely associated with it. Each lettered option may be selected once, more than once, or not at all.

Questions 183–186

   (A) Allo
   (B) Auto
   (C) Xeno
   (D) Iso

Match the following recipients of grafts with the correct prefix.

183. From self

184. From other species

185. From same species

186. From identical twins

Questions 187–192

    (A) ALG
    (B) Azathioprine
    (C) Cyclosporin
    (D) Methotrexate
    (E) OKT3
    (F) Steroid

Match the following mechanism of action associated with transplantation with the appropriate immunosuppressive agent.

187. Produces a decrease in total lymphocytes

188. Monoclonal antibody that binds to T_3 receptor

189. Purine analog that interferes with DNA synthesis

190. Inhibits T-cell activation and maturation

191. Folic acid antagonist that inhibits DNA and RNA synthesis

192. Sera directed against T lymphocytes

SURGERY ANSWERS AND DISCUSSION

1—A (Chapter 27) The main complication of total body hypothermia with a temperature of less than 30°C is cardiac arrhythmias. Total body hypothermia is defined as core temperature below 35°C and is classified as mild (32°C to 35°C), moderate (30°C to 32°C), or severe (below 30°C).

2—B (Chapter 19) At the time of diagnosis, cancer of the exocrine pancreas is confined to the pancreas in fewer than 10% of patients. In 75% of cases, pancreatic cancer occurs in the head of the pancreas. Approximately 75% of patients with pancreatic head carcinoma present with obstructive jaundice, weight loss (average, 20 lb), and deep-seated abdominal pain. A computed tomography (CT) scan should be ordered after baseline laboratory studies confirm an elevated bilirubin. A dynamic CT scan with fine cuts through the head of the pancreas often defines a mass in the head of the pancreas. Evidence of metastatic spread or involvement of the superior mesenteric artery can also be noted. These two features would deem the patient unresectable. Fine-needle aspiration (FNA) can be performed for accurate tissue diagnosis in patients who are not candidates for surgery. Endoscopic retrograde cholangiopancreatography (ERCP) is indicated for relief of biliary obstruction for those not resectable or if a definite mass is not seen on CT scan. In those patients determined preoperatively to be resectable, pancreatoduodenectomy (Whipple's resection) is the most commonly performed operation for carcinoma of the pancreatic head. Surgical palliation in patients with unresectable pancreatic carcinoma is directed toward relief of obstructive jaundice, gastric outlet obstruction, and pain. Malignant endocrine tumors are far less common than adenocarcinoma of the pancreas.

3—C (Chapter 1) Hemodynamic monitoring frequently reveals a high cardiac output *early* in the course of septic shock (hyperdynamic state). In 25% of cases, however, patients are found to have low cardiac output and high peripheral vascular resistance, consistent with a hypodynamic state. This latter group is indistinguishable from patients with hypovolemic shock. These two presentations probably represent a continuum of the same pathophysiology. The hypodynamic state is often seen late in the course when therapy has failed. Mortality rates from septic shock remain 50% to 70%. Cornerstones of therapy remain adequate surgical drainage of the septic focus, volume resuscitation, and appropriate antibiotic therapy.

4—D (Chapter 22) Closed loop obstruction results when both loops of the bowel are obstructed. This situation arises in cases such as volvulus, where the bowel loop is obstructed proximally and distally. Additionally, in a patient with a colonic obstruction with a competent ileocecal valve, there is a closed loop situation because material cannot leave from either end.

5—D (Chapter 2) Many hyponatremic states are asymptomatic until the sodium level falls below 120 mEq/L. An important exception is the patient with increased cerebrospinal pressure, such as following head injury in which mild hyponatremia may be deleterious or even fatal. Osmolality may increase, decrease, or remain unchanged in hyponatremia.

6—A (Chapter 24) Vigorous antibiotic treatment based on culture and sensitivity is considered the mainstay in the treatment of prostatitis. Sitz baths provide symptomatic relief but do not treat the condition per se.

7—C (Chapter 19) In acute pancreatitis, mortality rates of 50% are found with 5 to 6 signs identified as Ranson's criteria.

8—D (Chapter 5) *Staphylococcus aureus* usually is found in breast abscesses; however, breast abscesses may also be caused by gram-negative bacteria. These abscesses frequently occur in nursing mothers.

9—B (Chapter 5) The patient with a 3-cm laceration on the forearm caused by a rusty blade should receive tetanus immune globulin (TIG) and tetanus-diphtheria (Td) prophylaxis.

10—B (Chapter 1) Neurogenic shock follows a central failure of the autonomic nervous system to maintain peripheral vascular resistance, such as a high transection of the spinal cord.

11—B (Chapter 10) Tumors with no evidence of primary lesion present with lymph node metastases in approximately 3% to 4% of malignancies.

12—C (Chapter 5) A perirectal abscess is best treated by prompt incision and draining and antibiotic therapy. This abscess is caused by aerobic and anaerobic bacteria, which normally are found in the colon.

13—B (Chapter 1) The blood pressure is often low, but in contrast to other forms of shock, there is a *bradycardia* and the patient has warm, dry, or even flushed skin. In the management of these patients, the goal is to balance volume expansion with the risk of vasopressor administration.

14—A (Chapter 28) Fractures of the carpal scaphoid are prone to nonunion and aseptic necrosis of the proximal fragment because blood flows from distal to proximal and fractures disrupt this flow; therefore, the proximal segment becomes temporarily ischemic. Missed diagnosis and late treatment usually result in a high incidence of nonunion and aseptic necrosis of the proximal fragment.

15—C (Chapter 5) *Streptococcus pyogenes* is the most common organism that causes cellulitis, although organisms such as *Staphylococcus aureus*, *Streptococcus pneumoniae*, *Haemophilus influenzae*, and aerobic and anaerobic bacteria may be the cause.

16—C (Chapter 5) There is a single antivenin for all bites from pit vipers (antivenin *Crotalidae* polyvalent). In North America, all poisonous snakes of medical importance are members of the *Crotalidae* family (pit vipers).

17—C (Chapter 2) The maximum hourly administration of potassium to a patient with hypokalemia is 40 mEq/L in 1 hour with ECG monitoring.

18—D (Chapter 6) Normally, thromboxane A_2 activates platelets and causes aggregation; therefore, administering aspirin in low dosages causes inhibition of platelet production of thromboxane A_2, its principal mechanism of action as an anticoagulant.

19—A (Chapter 16) In a patient with transverse linear ecchymosis on the abdominal wall (seat-belt sign), the physician should be concerned about possible intestinal injury following blunt trauma.

20—D (Chapter 5) *Streptococcus pyogenes* most often causes erysipelas, a special type of cellulitis. This infection, in contrast to cellulitis, is characterized by a raised, sharply demarcated advancing margin.

21—B (Chapter 6, Table 6-1) Factors II, VII, IX, and X share the unique characteristic of having gamma carboxyl glutamic acid in their amino acid sequence, and they are dependent on vitamin K for activation. Without vitamin K, they do not undergo gamma carboxylation and are inactive.

22—B (Chapter 9) Organs can be successfully transplanted between identical twins without medication. Rejection occurs in all grafts except those between identical twins, acknowledging that individuals possess unique heritable differences in tissue histocompatibility antigens.

23—C (Chapter 11) Mammography is recommended for women between the ages of 40 and 50 years under the direction of a physician.

24—A (Chapter 5) A carbuncle is a subcutaneous abscess, which usually is formed by a confluent infection of multiple hair follicles. *Staphylococcus* is the most frequent microorganism cultured in this clinical setting.

25—D (Chapter 11) Lobular carcinoma *in situ* (LCIS) usually is not a component of progressive disease that leads to invasive lobular carcinoma. The presence of LCIS identifies patients that are at high risk for subsequently developing a breast cancer that is more often invasive ductal carcinoma; therefore, both breasts are at risk for cancer.

26—C (Chapter 1) Septic shock is an example of vasogenic shock, which is circulatory failure associated with a decrease in peripheral vascular resistance and an increase in central capacitance.

27—C (Chapter 10) The thyroid gland originates from the pharyngeal floor at the foramen cecum during the fourth week of gestation. It enlarges, becomes bilobed, and descends ventrally in the midline of the neck in close proximity to the hyoid bone. During its descent, the patent diverticulum is called the thyroglossal duct. The duct normally resorbs by the 10th week of gestation. When all or part of this duct persists, thyroglossal duct cysts or sinuses are formed. A thyroglossal duct cyst is not the same as a thyroid cyst, and thus it does not originate from the thyroid.

28–D (Chapter 10) Thyroglossal duct cysts generally are located in the midline of the neck in close proximity to the hyoid bone.

29–B (Chapter 5) Recommendations for tetanus prophylaxis with adsorbed tetanus toxoid require one injection followed by another in 4 to 6 weeks, and a third injection 6 to 12 months later.

30–B (Chapter 10) The antithyroid drug, propylthiouracil, is used initially in younger patients and in those who are pregnant or lactating in the treatment of hyperthyroidism.

31–A (Chapter 17) Gastric carcinoma commonly presents with symptoms suggestive of gastric ulcer.

32–D (Chapter 14) Ventricular septal defects are the most common congenital malformation of the heart, comprising 20% to 30% of all cases. Small defects should simply be observed because 60% to 70% close before the age of 3 years.

33–C (Chapter 10) When concerned with locoregional therapy for head and neck cancer, palliative procedures may produce relief of pain and airway obstruction or improvements in local function and hygiene, but they may also require the complete resection of local disease and may be justified even in the presence of distant disease.

34–D (Chapter 1) Shock is a clinical syndrome that results from tissue perfusion inadequate to maintain normal metabolic and nutritional activities. Although direct toxic factors may play a role in the development of shock, the common denominator in all forms of shock is reduced blood flow to vital organs.

35–C (Chapter 14) Right-to-left shunts of venous blood directly in the systemic circulation, producing arterial hypoxemia and cyanosis, result from the combination of intracardiac septal defect with obstruction to normal blood flow into the pulmonary artery. The classic example of this is tetralogy of Fallot (TOF), a combination of pulmonary stenosis and ventricular septal defect (VSD). Other cyanotic disorders include pulmonary stenosis-pulmonary atresia with intact ventricular septum, tricuspid atresia, truncus arteriosus, and transposition of the great vessels.

Cyanosis is the most prominent feature of right-to-left shunts. It is estimated that 5 g of reduced hemoglobin is required to produce cyanosis. Peripheral cyanosis results from a decrease in cardiac output and sluggish regional flow; central cyanosis results from a defect in oxygenation of blood in the lungs or an intracardiac shunt.

TOF is the most common cyanotic malformation. The four features of TOF are obstruction of the outflow tract of the right ventricle, a VSD, dextroposition of the aorta, and hypertrophy of the right ventricle. Anomalous coronary artery is found in 5% of patients.

Atrial septal defects (ASD), VSD, and patient ductus arteriosus (PDA) are examples of left-to-right shunts. Because pressures in the left atrium and left ventricle are normally greater than in the right atrium and right ventricle, a defect in the atrial or ventricular septum results in a shunt of oxygenated blood from the left side of the heart to the right side. This causes pulmonary congestion from an increase in pulmonary blood flow and often a corresponding decrease in systemic blood flow. Cyanosis does not occur.

36—C (Chapter 5) Tetanus is an infection usually caused by puncture wounds. The anaerobe, *Clostridium tetani*, is found in puncture wounds and in wounds with necrotic tissue and poor blood supply.

37—A (Chapter 10, Table 10-1) A typical presenting sign of thyrotoxicosis is atrial fibrillation. Common symptoms of thyrotoxicosis include weight loss, palpitations, heat intolerance and excessive sweating, emotional lability, and diarrhea. Signs seen frequently in addition to atrial fibrillation are warm smooth skin, tremor, proximal muscle weakness, widened pulse pressure with increased systolic and decreased diastolic pressures, and a hyperdynamic precordium with an accentuated S1. Constipation, low energy level, and hair loss on the outer third of the eyelid are common features of hypothyroidism.

38—C (Chapter 1) The Swan-Ganz catheter in the pulmonary artery, which monitors cardiac output and pulmonary artery pressures (including pulmonary artery wedge pressure and central venous pressure), is important in providing the basis for the appropriate volume of fluid administration.

39—A (Chapter 26) Varicose veins of the lower extremity are an extremely common affliction, affecting 15% to 20% of the population, with a female to male ratio of 5:1. They are classified as primary or secondary. Primary varicose veins are an isolated disorder of the superficial veins of the lower extremity and are not sequelae of deep venous thrombosis (DVT). Secondary varicosities are a manifestation of deep venous insufficiency and are associated with stigmata of chronic venous insufficiency, including edema, stasis dermatitis, skin pigmentation, ulceration, and the typical inflexible, scarred woody characteristic of the subcutaneous tissue.

40—C (Chapter 2) The first diagnostic or therapeutic maneuver in the patient with a potassium level of 7.3 mEq/L should be an ECG and administration of 1 g 10% calcium gluconate. This patient has hyperkalemia, and treatment should be directed at immediate cessation of exogenous administration of potassium, measures to stabilize the myocardium, and maneuvers to decrease serum potassium. Temporary suppression of the myocardium effects of a sudden rapid rise in potassium can be accomplished by the intravenous administration of 1 g of 10% calcium gluconate under ECG monitoring.

41—C (Chapter 3) Wound healing is characterized by inflammation, fibroplasia, and maturation. The steps overlap broadly, and the process is a continuum rather than a series of discrete changes.

42—A (Chapter 5) Current recommendations regarding preoperative antibiotic prophylaxis indicate that they should be given as a single dose 1 hour before surgery. This assures that peak drug levels are coincident with the time of incision. Generally, postoperative antibiotics are not recommended, although many surgeons administer one or two doses postoperatively.

43—C (Chapter 7) The most frequent serious complication directly attributable to transfusion is the transmission of disease, the most important of which is hepatitis. Hepatitis C is the most serious of the hepatitides because the risk of chronic active hepatitis is higher in hepatitis C than in hepatitis B. Human immunodeficiency virus (HIV) is routinely screened, and the risk today is minimal. Although ABO compatibility is a serious risk, transfusion reactions are usually the result of clerical error.

44—D (Chapter 1) Resuscitation is centered around replacement of intravascular volume and cessation of the source of intravascular fluid loss. Initially, crystalloids are used to increase the intravascular volume. If there is continued hypotension from ongoing blood loss, type-specific blood should be administered. In those cases in which there is insufficient time to obtain type-specific blood, O-negative blood is used. In the clinical setting of ongoing hypotension in a patient who has received massive amounts of crystalloids and colloid solutions, invasive monitors can be used to assess resuscitative efforts.

45—D (Chapter 25) During the first trimester of fetal life, precursor melanocytes arise from the neural crest and migrate to the skin, meninges, mucous membranes, upper esophagus, and eyes. In each of these locations they have demonstrated the potential for malignant transformation.

46—C (Chapter 19) Cullen's sign is ecchymotic discoloration around the umbilicus, caused by tracking of blood-stained fluid from the retroperitoneum along the falciform ligament. Retroperitoneal fluid tracking laterally causes an ecchymotic discoloration on the flanks. Caput Medusae is engorgement of periumbilical veins, associated with portal hypertension. Courvoisier's sign is the finding of a palpable dilated gallbladder, suggesting a pancreatic malignancy causing common duct obstruction.

47—C (Chapter 6) Warfarin impairs the formation of vitamin K-dependent factors by reducing the amount of vitamin K available for gamma carboxylation. Clinically, warfarin is followed by observing the prothrombin time (PT). Reversal of the effect of warfarin is by administration of vitamin K or by intravenous administration of coagulation factors.

48—C (Chapter 27) An insensate burn appears dry, dark, and leathery and is known as a third-degree burn, or a full-thickness burn. The skin also may appear translucent and mottled or waxy white. The surface is painless and generally dry.

49—C (Chapter 12) A ruptured emphysematous bleb is the most common cause of spontaneous pneumothorax.

50—A (Chapter 18) Chronic cholecystitis is characterized by intermittent, recurrent attacks of right upper quadrant pain and usually occurs approximately 30 to 60 minutes after eating a fatty or protein-rich meal. The pain lasts for several hours and then resolves.

51—B (Chapter 3) There is no appreciable increase in collagen content 21 days after wounding; therefore, collagen accumulation is maximal by this time. Wound strength increases significantly over the first 6 weeks after injury and then only slightly over the first 2 years.

52—D (Chapter 8) The most important aspect of total parenteral nutrition (TPN) is that parameters and a goal for the TPN regimen should be established before the initiation of TPN. The indications for TPN are broad and encompass a wide range of clinical situations ranging from newborns with catastrophic gastrointestinal anomalies to adults with sepsis syndrome.

53—C (Chapter 2) The osmolality of the serum is approximately 300 mOsm/L.

54—C (Chapter 7) In starving patients, oxygen consumption and metabolic rate are typically reduced, and caloric requirements decline over several weeks to months. The reduced energy requirements are met by mobilization of fat, and a certain level of obligatory skeletal muscle breakdown occurs to support gluconeogenesis.

55—C (Chapter 2) The sodium deficit can be calculated by multiplying the deficit of serum sodium below normal (in mEq/L) by the liters of *total body water*. Note that the estimate is based on total body water, since the effective osmotic pressure in the extracellular compartment cannot be increased without increasing this fraction proportionally in the intracellular compartment. In this patient, the sodium deficit is calculated as follows:

[Normal saline (mEq/L) – measured sodium (mEq/L)]
    × total body water = Deficit (mEq)
140 – 120 × 70 × 60% = 20 × 42 = 840 mEq

56—D (Chapter 2) Generally, only a portion of the total deficit is replaced initially to relieve acute symptoms. Further correction is facilitated when renal function is restored by correction of the volume deficit. Of importance, central pontine and extrapontine myelinolysis may occur with rapid correction of hyponatremia and may cause irreversible central nervous system (CNS) damage or death. It is recommended, therefore, that the serum sodium level not be increased more than 12 mEq/L during the first 24 hours, and even less during each subsequent 24-hour period.

57—D (Chapter 7) There is no basis for transfusion based on a hematocrit value. However, it is well accepted that continuing hemorrhage requires transfusion of red blood cells eventually. As red blood cells are lost, there is a diminishing capacity of the blood to carry oxygen. Under proper circumstances, anemia down to half the normal level of hematocrit can be well tolerated (20 to 25 mg/dL). Patients who are stable should be allowed to replace their own red blood cell mass. Favoring transfusion for anemia are conditions in which the patient may soon face increased demands or *further* significant blood loss, or in which there are preexisting disorders, especially coronary atherosclerosis, which make anemia less well tolerated.

58—D (Chapter 26) A ventilation/perfusion (V/Q) scan would be the next test to document a pulmonary embolism. When the V/Q scan shows intermediate probability for a pulmonary embolism, a pulmonary angiogram should be obtained.

59—D (Chapter 18) Choledocholithiasis implies the presence of gallstones in the common bile duct and can be associated with ascending cholangitis. This disease manifests clinically as jaundice. Many patients have associated right upper quadrant pain and fever.

60—E (Chapter 2) Total body water is divided into two compartments. The fluid within the body's diverse cell population, *intracellular water*, represents 60% to 70% of total body water, or 30% to 40% of total body weight. The *extracellular water* represents approximately 25% to 35% of total body water, or 20% of total body weight; this compartment is subdivided into the *intravascular fluid*, or plasma (5% of total body weight), and the *interstitial fluid* (15% of total body weight). Following local trauma or diffuse body injury, there is an internal loss of extracellular fluid into a **nonfunctional** space (third space), such as sequestration of isotonic fluid in a burn, peritonitis, ascites, or muscle trauma. Interstitial fluid and third-space fluid loss are *not* synonymous terms.

61—B (Chapter 9) The major histocompatibility complex (MHC) is located on chromosome 6. In humans, the gene products of the MHC were first investigated on leukocytes and were called human leukocyte antigens (HLA).

62—A (Chapter 12) This condition most commonly results from penetrating injuries. The human pericardial sac is a fibrous fixed structure, and only a relatively small amount of blood is required to restrict cardiac activity and interfere with cardiac filling. The classic Beck's triad consists of elevated venous pressure, decreased arterial pressure, and muffled heart tones. Pulsus paradoxus, a decrease in systolic pressure during inspiration in excess of 10 mm Hg, and Kussmaul's sign, a rise in venous pressure with inspiration, may also be present. Pericardiocentesis is the indicated treatment; removal of as little as 15 to 20 mL blood or fluid may result in immediate hemodynamic improvement.

63—D (Chapter 16, Table 16-1) Injuries to the retroperitoneum are difficult to diagnose because this area is remote from physical examination and is not assessed by diagnostic peritoneal lavage (DPL).

64—A (Chapter 20) Postsplenectomy sepsis is most commonly found in children younger than 4 years of age and within 2 years after splenectomy. It accounts for 80% of cases. Following splenectomy, the risk of overwhelming infections is approximately 60 times greater than normal and may be as high as 0.5% to 1.9% yearly.

65—C (Chapter 6) Fresh frozen plasma (FFP) is the only source of factor V. Factor V is present in plasma but not in serum.

66—B (Chapter 11) Fibroadenomas of the breast occur primarily in females who are in their second or third decade of life.

67—D (Chapter 10) In the United States, the most common form of carcinoma of the thyroid is papillary carcinoma.

68—C (Chapter 13) Pulmonary sequestration is a condition in which a portion of the lung is isolated from the remainder of the lung during development and receives its blood supply from an aberrant branch of the aorta instead of the pulmonary artery. The sequestered lobe is prone to develop recurrent infections.

69—C (Chapter 5) Deaths following bites from rattlesnakes account for most snakebite-related deaths (70%) in the United States.

70—B (Chapter 14) Current indications for coronary artery bypass grafting include patients with mild angina but with left main coronary artery disease. Other indications include patients with triple vessel disease and depressed myocardial function, those with moderate to severe angina not responding to medical management, those with unstable angina, those with acute infarction demonstrating evidence of subendocardial infarction, hemodynamic instability, and postinfarction patients with left main artery disease or triple vessel disease.

71—C (Chapter 2) The extracellular fluid represents 25% to 35% of total body water.

72—A (Chapter 11) Gynecomastia implies the presence of a female-type mammary gland in a male. It can be induced by anabolic steroids. Gynecomastia occurs most often during three phases of life: the neonatal period, adolescence, or senescence. It does not predispose to male breast cancer, nor is total mastectomy a treatment of choice in managing this disease.

73—B (Chapter 2) Overadministration of diuretics is associated with chloride-responsive metabolic acidosis. This type of metabolic alkalosis is associated with extracellular volume deficits (especially following diuretic therapy).

74—B (Chapter 5) Rabies is best treated with vaccine prophylaxis in appropriate cases. The circumstances surrounding the bite often provide clues as to whether a vaccine is indicated; an unprovoked attack by a domestic animal or exposure to dogs outside the United States would most likely be treated best with vaccine prophylaxis.

75—D (Chapter 10) The normal volume of salivary secretion in men ranges from 1000 to 1500 mL daily. This secretion is primarily in the form of serous fluid from the parotid and submandibular glands.

76—D (Chapter 25) Keratoacanthoma is a benign lesion of the skin that must be differentiated from squamous cell carcinoma. Keratoacanthomas are characterized by rapid growth, often reaching full size within a few weeks. They usually are seen on older persons as a single lesion. They are 1 to 2 cm in diameter, with a characteristic horn-filled crater. The lesion is biopsied to establish diagnosis.

77—B (Chapter 2) If extracellular osmolality is reduced too rapidly, convulsions and coma may result as water shifts into brain cells. For this reason, correction of hypernatremia is best accomplished with administration of half-strength balanced saline solution. In the absence of a significant volume deficit, water (D_5W) should be administered cautiously because hypervolemia may result.

78—C (Chapter 3) Full-thickness skin grafts are the most effective way to control wound contracture.

79—C (Chapter 2) Addition of isotonic saline solution to the intravascular space results in an increase in extracellular volume.

80—B (Chapter 28) In fat embolism syndrome, droplets of fat from the bone marrow enter the systemic circulation and impair pulmonary capillary perfusion by a complex mechanism. Fat droplets occasionally are visible in blood specimens and in urine.

81—A (Chapter 6) Cryoprecipitate is the best source of fibrinogen and of factor VIII and von Willebrand's factor. The major advantages to using cryoprecipitate are its small volume and single-donor status.

82—C (Chapter 3) Macrophages are essential to wound healing. They appear to be the prime factor in regulating collagen elaboration by the fibroblasts.

83—E (Chapter 10) Men older than 40 years of age with a history of tobacco and alcohol use comprise 70% to 80% of most patients with head and neck cancer. Symptoms referable to the tumor itself are usually mild and not commensurate with the size of the tumor. Late-stage presentation is common in these patients, which accounts for the high mortality rate.

84—C (Chapter 22) For the patient with Dukes' stage C colon cancer, postoperative chemoradiation therapy is recommended. Dukes' stage C1 classification indicates invasion to the serosa with lymph node metastases; stage C2 indicates invasion of the pericolonic fat and lymph node metastases.

85–D (Chapter 19) Pseudocysts are localized collections of fluid with high concentrations of pancreatic enzymes. They usually occur as a complication of pancreatitis. They are located either within the parenchyma or in one of the potential spaces that separate the gland from the adjacent abdominal viscera. Most often they are found in the lesser sac behind the stomach. If mature pseudocysts are less than 5 cm in diameter, they most likely do not require treatment; however, they should be followed by serial ultrasound. Cysts requiring operative intervention are usually drained internally, although external drainage and excision are other options. A portion of the wall should always be biopsied to exclude a diagnosis of cystadenocarcinoma of the pancreas.

86–B (Chapter 10) The majority of salivary gland tumors are present in the parotid gland. Of tumors of the parotid gland, 80% are benign; most (80%) are classified as pleomorphic adenomas.

87–A (Chapter 3) Polymorphonuclear lymphocytes act to phagocytize bacteria from the wound in the process of healing.

88–A (Chapter 5) A felon is a purulent collection in the distal phalanx of the finger and causes intense pain and pressure in that compartment.

89–C (Chapter 11) Mammography should *not* be used as a substitute for biopsy but as an adjunctive complementary study that augments history and physical examination.

90–A (Chapter 10) The parotid gland drains into the mouth via Stensen's duct.

91–B (Chapter 11) In the United States, breast cancer is the second leading cause of death from cancer in women. It is second to lung cancer.

92–C (Chapter 10) The hallmark of Riedel's thyroiditis is a woody, hard thyroid caused by fibrosis, which usually extends into surrounding neck structures. It is also known as invasive fibrous thyroiditis.

93–A (Chapter 24) Transillumination of the scrotum may help confirm the diagnosis of hydrocele, which is a cystic enlargement of the tunica vaginalis. This condition is frequently asymptomatic, except for the presence of a mass. Aspiration yields clear fluid. Treatment of choice is surgical excision by opening the sac and everting it about the testicle.

94–B (Chapter 11) Fine-needle aspiration (FNA) can establish the diagnosis of breast cancer in a patient with a palpable mass.

95–C (Chapter 25) Nodular melanoma is classified as a subjunctional melanoma, which usually demonstrates a predominant vertical growth phase and, therefore, very early metastases.

96–A (Chapter 11) Paget's disease of the breast is best characterized as a chronic eczematous eruption of the nipple.

97—C (Chapter 17) Operations for duodenal ulcers are aimed at decreasing gastric acid production and include truncal vagotomy, highly selective vagotomy, and removal of the gastric antrum. The operation with the lowest risk of recurring ulcers is the truncal vagotomy and antrectomy.

98—A (Chapter 11) Carcinoma of the breast occurs in one of eight women in the United States. Except on rare occasions, the presenting symptom is a painless lump that has developed insidiously. It is rare for patients with early invasive breast cancer to have clinically detectable distant metastases at the time of initial diagnosis.

99—B (Chapter 12) A flail chest occurs when a segment of the chest wall does not have bony continuity with the remainder of the thoracic cage. This condition results from trauma associated with multiple rib fractures. The major difficulty in flail chest stems from the injury to the underlying lung parenchyma; the defect in the chest wall alone does not cause hypoxemia. Initial therapy includes adequate ventilation, administration of humidified oxygen, and careful fluid resuscitation.

100—D (Chapter 11) Fibroadenomas of the breast sometimes present with concurrent lobular carcinoma *in situ*. Fibroadenomas have a relationship with estrogen sensitivity and occur predominantly during the second and third decades of life.

101—A (Chapter 10) Hashimoto's disease, or chronic lymphocytic or autoimmune thyroiditis, is one of the most common autoimmune diseases. It is the most common cause of hypothyroidism.

102—A (Chapter 13) Lung abscesses are most commonly caused by aspiration; treatment consists of antibiotics and drainage. High doses of antibiotics are administered intravenously based on sensitivities of the infecting organism. Spontaneous drainage by expectoration is adequate in most cases.

103—B (Chapter 24) Nephrolithiasis (or renal calculi) affects approximately 1% to 3% of the adult population. More than 90% of stones are radiopaque. Because of advances in fiber optics and the subsequent development of small-caliber flexible instruments and extracorporeal shock wave lithotripsy, which has led to a decrease in open procedures, most patients with renal calculi do not require surgery.

104—C (Chapter 24) Benign prostatic hypertrophy (BPH) can have a significant impact on quality of life. It is the most common disorder of the prostate gland. Symptoms include frequent urination, decreased force of urine stream, hesitation in the initiation of flow, intermittency, a sensation of incomplete emptying, and nocturia to a variable degree. By age 80 years, 90% of men have histologic evidence of BPH.

105—C (Chapter 10) Medullary carcinoma of the thyroid is a C-cell calcitonin-producing tumor and occurs in families as part of the multiple endocrine neoplasia type II (MEN-II) syndrome.

106—C (Chapter 11) Fine-needle aspiration (FNA) can be used for nonpalpable masses detected by mammography. In most centers, the false-negative interpretation is less than 10%; false-positives are rare.

107—B (Chapter 5) Rates of wound infections in clean wounds tend to be approximately 2%.

108—D (Chapter 15) The most accurate way to diagnose gastro-esophageal reflux disease (GERD) is by measuring the number of hours the pH is less than 4 during a 24-hour period.

109—B (Chapter 25) The current risk of melanoma in the white population is approximately 1 in 150.

110—C (Chapter 19) The most common cause of acute pancreatitis in the United States is gallstones (cholelithiasis).

111—C (Chapter 5) The rate of infection for a contaminated wound is approximately 8.5%.

112—A (Chapter 28) The most common shoulder dislocation is the traumatic anterior dislocation of the shoulder. The cumulative range of motion of the shoulder is greater than any other joint because of the lack of bony and soft tissue constraints.

113—C (Chapter 11) The best treatment option for patients with lobular carcinoma *in situ* is lifelong observation of both breasts with mammography and physical examination.

114—A (Chapter 16) The only contraindication to diagnostic peritoneal lavage (DPL) or computed tomography (CT) is when the patient has a pressing need for exploratory laparotomy for celiotomy.

115—C (Chapter 18) Cholelithiasis denotes the presence of stones in the gallbladder but does not imply disease. It is chronic and usually occurs more often in women than in men. Cholelithiasis is frequently subject to acute exacerbations causing biliary colic. Gallstone formation is thought to result from abnormalities in the composition of bile.

116—C (Chapter 25) The Breslow level associated with an almost 90% cure rate with simple excision alone in malignant melanoma is thickness of less than 0.76 mm.

117—A (Chapter 22) Obstruction of the orifice of the appendix causes a closed loop obstruction. There is continued normal appendiceal secretions, which are unable to leave the appendix because of the obstruction. These secretions, together with rapid bacterial overgrowth within the appendiceal lumen, result in increased intraluminal pressure. The increased pressure causes distention and results in decreased mucosal blood flow, causing ulceration of the mucosa. The inflammation and infection spreads throughout the wall of the appendix, and the appendiceal wall rapidly becomes gangrenous and necrotic. If unattended, perforation can result.

118—D (Chapter 12) The most common anterior mediastinal mass is a thymoma, with operative intervention almost always indicated to provide definitive diagnosis and simultaneously provide information toward definitive treatment.

119—C (Chapter 19) The predominant clinical feature of acute pancreatitis is penetrating epigastric pain, radiating to the back. Other features include elevated concentrations of pancreatic enzymes in blood and an increased amount of pancreatic enzyme in the urine.

120—A (Chapter 28) The treatment of choice for hip fractures is open reduction and internal fixation. Hip fractures are most common in elderly women.

121—C (Chapter 22) Inguinal hernias are the most common hernia in women, just as they are in men. Femoral hernias are more common in women than in men, but in absolute numbers. Inguinal hernias in women outnumber femoral hernias.

122—A (Chapter 19) Alcoholism is the most common cause of chronic pancreatitis in the United States.

123—A (Chapter 21) Esophageal varices result from portosystemic anastomoses between the left gastric vein. The most important natural portosystemic anastomoses is between the left gastric or coronary vein, which joins the splenic or portal vein near its confluence and connects with the esophageal venous plexus and also with the tributaries of the superior vena cava.

124—C (Chapter 22) Right-sided colon cancers frequently have metastasized by the time of physical examination. Diagnosis is often suspected on history, and physical examination may reveal a palpable mass on rectal examination or occult blood in the stool.

125—D (Chapter 22) Crohn's disease has transmural involvement microscopically, whereas disease is limited to the mucosa in ulcerative colitis.

126—B (Chapter 18) Acute cholecystitis is characterized by acute inflammation of the gallbladder and usually associated with bacterial infection. Attacks usually occur at night and often follow a dietary indiscretion such as overeating. Pain is severe and presents in the epigastrium or right upper quadrant, frequently radiating to the back, scapular region, or right shoulder.

127—B (Chapter 5) The patient should receive a diphtheria-pertussis-tetanus (DPT) shot.

128—D (Chapter 28) Fractures of the clavicle occur most often in children younger than age 10 years. Most of these fractures require only symptomatic treatment, with support for the shoulder and arm provided by a stockinette bandage. These fractures usually do not cause injury to surrounding structures.

129—D (Chapter 20) *Streptococcus pneumoniae* accounts for postsplenectomy infection in more than 50% of cases. Other common offending organisms include *Neisseria meningitidis, Escherichia coli,* and *Haemophilus influenzae.*

130—B (Chapter 22) Only 20% of patients with partial small bowel obstruction eventually require operative intervention. These patients are those whose small bowel obstruction is 2% adhesions.

131—D (Chapter 28) Intravenous antibiotics are not necessary in the treatment of a closed fracture. They are given before surgery when treating an open fracture.

132—A (Chapter 23) A total of 10% of pheochromocytomas are bilateral, 10% are extraadrenal, and 10% are malignant. Pheochromocytomas are endocrine tumors of the adrenal medulla and produce norepinephrine and epinephrine. The chief symptom is sustained diastolic hypertension and paroxysmal hypertensive episodes.

133—B (Chapter 5) A common bile duct exploration for ascending cholangitis is not an example of a clean-contaminated wound. In clean-contaminated wounds, contamination may arise from the skin and an opening in the biliary tract, gastrointestinal tract (including appropriately prepared large bowel), or respiratory tree. Contaminated wounds, such as that described in B, are those in which there is an open, fresh traumatic wound, entrance of biliary and genitourinary tracts in the presence of infected bile or urine, a major break in technique, or an incision in which acute nonpurulent inflammation is present.

134—B (Chapter 22) Carcinoid tumors in the small intestine produce carcinoid syndrome *with metastases* to the liver. These tumors metastasize with greater frequency than carcinoids elsewhere in the gastrointestinal tract.

135—B (Chapter 2) *Total body water* constitutes between 50% and 70% of total body weight. The average normal value is 60% of body weight for young adult men and 50% for young adult women. Fat contains less water; therefore, an obese patient has less body water than a lean individual, and females who on average have a higher percentage of total body fat have less body water than males. Total body water also decreases with increasing age.

136—C (Chapter 10) Late-stage presentation of head and neck cancer is common (*not uncommon*) because symptoms referable to the tumor are mild. These patients, therefore, usually do not present until the cancer is in later stages, which relates to the high incidence and mortality rates in the United States.

137—C (Chapter 12) Distant heart sounds would not suggest the diagnosis of right-sided tension pneumothorax. Tension pneumothorax is characterized by respiratory distress, tachycardia, hypotension, tracheal deviation, unilateral absence of breath sounds, neck vein distention, and cyanosis as a late manifestation.

138—B (Chapter 4) There is most likely no justification in modern practice for the routine placement of an open drain in a clean or clean-contaminated surgical wound. Previously, it was advocated that these drains be placed in the subhepatic space following bowel anastomoses and in the perineum following abdominoperineal resections. Today, the widespread use of prophylactic antibiotics in surgery has gradually displaced the prophylactic use of drains. There seems to be little reason to insert drains solely to prevent infection, particularly when prophylactic antibiotics are administered concurrently.

139—D (Chapter 28) Pulselessness is *not* an early clinical manifestation of compartment syndrome, although it is a *later* manifestation of this syndrome. Compartment syndrome is a serious complication following extremity trauma or ischemic injury, where pain is an early sign; blood pressures of 30 to 40 mm Hg are an indication for fasciotomy.

140—D (Chapter 15) Esophageal cancer should be suspected in a patient with a history of smoking, columnar metaplasia, and weight loss of 35 lb in the past year. The most common cause of dysphagia is cancer of the esophagus. Midsternal chest pain is *not* a likely symptom of esophageal cancer.

141—C (Chapter 12) Murphy's sign is not associated with cardiac tamponade. All of the following may be present: Beck's triad, consisting of elevated venous pressure, decreased arterial pressure, and muffled heart tones; pulsus paradoxus, a decrease in systolic pressure during inspiration in excess of 10 mm Hg; and Kussmaul's sign, a rise in venous pressure with inspiration.

142—A (Chapter 21, Table 21-1) An increase in alanine aminotransferase (ALT) does not imply cholestasis. It usually implies hepatocyte damage.

143—E (Chapter 10) Albumin, amylase, immunoglobulins A, G, and M, and lysozyme are all substances secreted in saliva. Trypsin is a serine endopeptidase that is secreted by the pancreas and is important to protein digestion; it is not secreted in saliva.

144—B (Chapter 8) In those patients unable to take adequate oral alimentation but have a functioning gastrointestinal tract, the preferred method of addressing their nutritional deficiency is by *enteral feeds*. Nasogastric feeding should *only* be used in alert patients because the risk of aspiration is high in those patients who are unable to protect their airways. Not all patients who are off ventilators can protect their airways. A nasoduodenal tube with continuous infusion pumps is a better option in these patients. Percutaneously endoscopically placed gastrostomy (PEG) tubes are a good method of feeding patients with lesions arising above the level of the gastroesophageal junction. Gastrostomy feeding is contraindicated in mentally obtunded patients.

145—D (Chapter 5) The appropriate treatment of cellulitis consists of antibiotics, local application of heat, adequate immobilization, and elevation of the affected extremity. Incision and drainage are *not used* in the management of cellulitis.

146—A (Chapter 10) Parathyroid hormone (PTH) level is increased in primary, secondary, and tertiary hyperparathyroidism.

147—D (Chapter 10) In the United States, solitary nodules are clinically present in 4% to 6% of patients. Cancer of the thyroid occurs with an incidence of 50 new cases per million population in this country (approximately 12,000 new cases per year). By far, most thyroid nodules are benign; males have fewer benign lesions than females. Previous radiation exposure and age older than 40 years in men or older than 50 years in women increase the likelihood of malignancy. Scintillation scanning localizes the site of radioactive iodine (^{123}I) or ^{99m}Tc pertechnetate. Nodules in the thyroid can be hyperfunctional or hypofunctional. Most carcinomas present as "cold" nodules. Fine-needle aspiration of the nodule should follow. All patients with malignant cytology should undergo operation. All patients with sheets of follicular cells should undergo operation; follicular cancers exhibit the same cytology as follicular adenomas and cannot be differentiated by this technique.

148—B (Chapter 15) It is *not* necessary to ascertain the presence of esophagitis by endoscopy before surgical intervention for gastroesophageal reflux disease (GERD) is attempted. Demonstration of a defective lower esophageal sphincter mechanism, increased esophageal exposure to gastric juice on a 24-hour pH study, and presence of adequate esophageal contractions are necessary to ascertain before surgical intervention for GERD.

149—A (Chapter 18) *Bacteroides fragilis* is the only organism of those listed that is *not* commonly found in the bile of patients with acute cholecystitis. Agents commonly isolated include *Enterococcus*, *Escherichia coli*, and *Klebsiella*.

150—B (Chapter 3) The type of suture material used influences wound healing because all sutures are foreign bodies and none used clinically are devoid of tissue reaction. Metal sutures are *not* devoid of tissue reaction; they stimulate minimal response in tissues. The suture material selected is based on characteristics of the suture, preferences of the surgeon, suture availability, and tissue to be sutured.

151—A (Chapter 5) Contact with the blood, urine, or feces of a rabid animal does not constitute exposure, and prophylaxis is not indicated for this patient.

152—B (Chapter 22) Major causes of small bowel obstruction include adhesions, hernias, and malignant tumors; gallstone ileus is not one of the major causes of small bowel obstruction.

153—D (Chapter 6) Heparin is an anticoagulant used clinically. It inhibits coagulation by forming a complex with antithrombin III (AT III). This complex inactivates thrombin (IIa) and factors VII, IX, X, and XI. Clinically, the effect of heparin is followed by measuring the PTT or aPTT. Addition of fresh frozen plasma (FFP) does *not* reverse the action of heparin; because the clotting factors in FFP are transfused, they are inactivated by the circulating heparin. The effect of heparin can be reversed by administration of protamine.

154—D (Chapter 11) No studies have shown that there is increased risk of breast cancer in patients with fibrocystic breast disease. *Most lesions are not risk factors*; however, if there is associated dysplasia, the risk of breast cancer increases.

155—D (Chapter 2) If acidosis is due to a loss of bicarbonate (as in pancreatic fistula) or a gain of chloride, the anion gap is normal. Conversely, if the acidosis is due to the increased production of an organic acid (lactate in shock, ketoacids in starvation) or the retention of a sulfuric or phosphoric acid (as in renal failure), then the anion gap increases.

156—C (Chapter 17) In patients with dumping syndrome, vomiting is not a common characteristic. Dumping syndrome is characterized by feelings of faintness, sweating, palpitations, and nausea shortly after eating. Treatment is aimed at increasing intake of fat, decreasing carbohydrates, and liquids are given between meals.

157—B (Chapter 26) Operative indications for peripheral vascular disease fall into one of four broad categories: (1) limb salvage: surgical revascularization can prevent limb loss secondary to gangrene and ischemic ulceration; (2) limb salvage: surgical thromboembolectomy to reestablish blood flow to an extremity; (3) intolerable rest pain: surgical revascularization to decrease symptomatology; and (4) preservation of function such as radiologic or surgical intervention to treat disabling claudication, which limits self-care, occupation, or desired recreation. In patients with new onset claudication, measures such as cessation of tobacco products and an exercise program decrease claudication without the need for surgical/radiologic intervention.

158—B (Chapter 24) Urinary catheters are sensitive indicators of volume status of the patient. However, a urethral catheter should not be placed in a patient in whom urethral transection is suspected. Urethral injury should be suspected if there is blood in the penile (urethral) meatus, blood in the scrotum or ecchymosis of the scrotum, or the prostate is high riding or cannot be palpated on rectal examination. Accordingly, urethral catheterization should not be attempted before an examination of the rectum and external genitalia has been performed.

159—A (Chapter 5, Table 5-3) The decision for prophylaxis is based on the severity of the wound and the availability of the animal for observation and autopsy to substantiate the diagnosis of rabies. Postexposure prophylaxis in addition to local wound care consists of human rabies immune globulin (HRIG) and vaccine (HRIG is *always* given; this is in contrast to tetanus immune globulin (TIG), which is given selectively).

Currently, there are two rabies vaccines available: human diploid cell rabies vaccine (HDCV) and rabies vaccine adsorbed (RVA). Either is administered in conjunction *with* HRIG at the beginning of postexposure prophylaxis. The first dose is given as soon as possible after exposure. Additional doses are given on days 3, 7, 14, and 28 after the initial injection. For adults, the *vaccine* is always given in the *deltoid* area, whereas the anterolateral aspect of the thigh is acceptable for children. Injection of RVA or HDCV in the gluteal region should never be used because it results in lower neutralizing antibody titers. *HRIG* is administered only once (20 IU/kg) and is injected in the *gluteal* region.

Human rabies immune globulin (HRIG) is given as postexposure prophylaxis in addition to local wound care.

160—D (Chapter 3) Collagen synthesis and wound healing are suppressed by decreased PO_2 in the healing tissues and low blood flow and, additionally, deficiency of vitamin C and hyperglycemia (associated with diabetes mellitus).

161—D (Chapter 22) Complications of diverticular disease of the colon include bleeding, obstruction, and perforation; perianal fistula is *not* a complication of diverticular disease. Diverticular disease indicates the presence of colonic diverticula, a condition that is rare before the age of 30 years but becomes more common with increasing age.

162—D (Chapter 9) Transplantation of heart, lungs, kidneys, liver, and pancreas have all been successful.

163—D (Chapter 13) Bronchogenic carcinoma is divided into two groups: small cell lung cancer (SCLC) and non-small cell lung cancer (NSCLC); untreated SCLC has the most rapidly adverse clinical course of any type of pulmonary tumor, with a median survival time from time of diagnosis of only 2 to 4 months.

164—D (Chapter 10) Papillary carcinoma is the least invasive of the carcinomas of the thyroid. In the United States, papillary carcinoma comprises two-thirds of all thyroid cancers, follicular represents 18%, medullary less than 10%, and anaplastic 10% to 15%.

165—B (Chapter 10) Thyrotoxicosis refers to a spectrum of clinical manifestations that are related to excessive secretion of active thyroid hormone. The three primary types of pathologic processes associated with thyrotoxicosis are Graves' disease, toxic adenoma, and toxic multinodular goiter. It is *not* associated with Riedel's thyroiditis, which is extremely rare and of unknown etiology.

166—C (Chapter 10) Parathyroid hormone (PTH) is essential for calcium homeostasis. PTH affects bone and kidney primarily. In the bone, it stimulates calcium resorption; in the kidney, it significantly increases the resorption of calcium and 1-hydroxylation of 25-hydroxyvitamin D_3, which in turn enhances intestinal absorption of calcium and phosphates. Release of PTH by the parathyroid glands is through a negative feedback system. A *fall* in serum calcium (or serum magnesium) concentration stimulates secretion of PTH; an elevation of serum calcium *reduces* both serum PTH and formation of 1,25-hydroxyvitamin D_3.

167—D (Chapter 26) Virchow's triad characterizes the pathophysiology of the formation of thrombi in the venous system and includes stasis of the blood in the veins, injury to the intimal surface of the veins (predisposing them to thrombosis), and a generalized state of hypercoagulability. Varicose veins are not a part of this triad.

168—B (Chapter 10) Medullary carcinoma of the thyroid is not associated with multiple endocrine neoplasia type I (MEN-I). Symptoms associated with MEN-I include hyperparathyroidism, pancreatic neoplasm, and pituitary neoplasm.

169—A (Chapter 13) A physician *would not* order a bone scan to determine the resectability of a lesion in the right upper lobe. Bronchoscopy, computed tomography (CT) of the chest, and pulmonary function tests would all be appropriate diagnostic tools.

170—C (Chapter 17) Night pain does not indicate a need for surgical intervention in the management of peptic ulcer disease. With the advent of H_2-receptor blockers and hydrogen potassium proton pump inhibitors, surgical therapy for peptic ulcer disease has diminished. However, gastric outlet obstruction, intractable bleeding, and perforated ulcer are indications for surgery.

171—C (Chapter 11) Lobular carcinoma *in situ* is not contraindicated in breast-conservation treatment. Contraindications to breast-conservation therapy include multifocal primary tumors, large tumor/breast-size ratio, collagen vascular disease, and lack of patient commitment to undergo irradiation and close follow-up.

172—A (Chapter 21) Features that characterize the liver include the following: it has a dual blood supply, enterohepatic circulation, and capacity to regenerate. It is not a center for acid-base control.

173—C (Chapter 10) Pleomorphic tumors occurs most frequently during the fifth decade with a slight *female* predominance.

174—A (Chapter 27) When a patient is admitted to the hospital after sustaining a burn injury, the physician should be alert to the possibility of airway involvement. Clinical indication of inhalation injury includes facial burns, singeing of the eyes and nasal vibrissae, carbon deposits and acute inflammatory changes in the oropharynx, carbonaceous sputum, history of impaired mentation, and history of explosion or fire in a closed environment.

175—C (Chapter 3) Silk is not an absorbable suture. Nonabsorbable sutures act as foreign bodies and perpetuate the infection until extruded or removed. Nonabsorbable sutures are subcategorized as monofilament or braided, or synthetic or natural.

176—D (Chapter 15) There are three normal areas of esophageal narrowing. The uppermost narrowing is located at the entrance into the esophagus and is caused by the cricopharyngeal muscle. It is the narrowest point of the esophagus. The middle narrowing is due to an indentation of the anterior and left lateral esophageal wall, caused by the crossing of the left main-stem bronchus and aortic arch. The lowermost narrowing is at the diaphragmatic hiatus and is caused by the gastroesophageal sphincter mechanism. The indentation due to the right atrium is not a normal area of esophageal narrowing.

177—A (Chapter 19) Zollinger-Ellison syndrome is not characterized by the presence of ulcers and constipation.

178—B (Chapter 14) Hypertrophy of the left ventricle is not a feature of tetralogy of Fallot. The four features of tetralogy of Fallot include obstruction of the outflow tract of the right ventricle, a ventral septal defect, dextroposition of the aorta, and hypertrophy of the *right* ventricle.

179—C (Chapter 1) Massive blood loss is *not* a characteristic of cardiogenic shock. Cardiogenic shock is defined as circulatory failure caused by the inability of the heart to serve as an adequate pump. Arrhythmia, decreased cardiac output, and myocardial infarction are all characteristics of cardiogenic shock.

180—B (Chapter 22) Diarrhea is not a cardinal sign or symptom of intestinal obstruction. Abdominal distention, episodic abdominal pain, obstipation, and vomiting are indications of intestinal obstruction.

181—D (Chapter 24) The classic triad of pain, mass, and hematuria occurs late in renal cell carcinoma and is seen in less than 50% of patients. Although renal cell cancer can grow to occupy the inferior vena cava, lower body swelling is rare.

182—C (Chapter 3) Although neutrophils decrease infection, they are *not* essential to normal healing of sterile wounds. The second cell to make its appearance, the blood monocyte (called a macrophage after it leaves the circulation), is not only phagocytic but is of central importance in regulating subsequent cellular activities in the wound healing process. Collagen synthesis and wound healing are suppressed by decreased PO_2 in the healing tissues and low blood flow and, additionally, deficiency of vitamin C, diabetes, liver insufficiency, renal insufficiency (uremia), distant malignancies, and administration of corticosteroids impair wound healing. The impairment caused by corticosteroids can be mitigated by administration of vitamin A.

183—B (Chapter 9) Autografts are grafts from individuals to themselves. These transplants survive indefinitely after the vascular supply has been reestablished.

184—C (Chapter 9) Grafts between individuals of different species are known as xenografts, or heterografts. They are rejected quite rapidly.

185—A (Chapter 9) Grafts between the same species are known as allografts and are rejected greatly in proportion to the degree of genetic disparity between the donor and the recipient.

186—D (Chapter 9) Grafts between identical twins are known as isografts. Like autografts, these grafts survive indefinitely after the vascular supply has been reestablished.

187—F (Chapter 9, Table 9-1) Steroids produce a decrease in total lymphocytes.

188—E (Chapter 9, Table 9-1) OKT3 is a monoclonal antibody that binds to the T_3 receptor.

189—B (Chapter 9, Table 9-1) Azathioprine is a purine analog that interferes with DNA synthesis.

190—C (Chapter 9, Table 9-1) Cyclosporin inhibits T-cell activation and maturation.

191—D (Chapter 9, Table 9-1) Methotrexate is a folic acid antagonist that inhibits DNA and RNA synthesis.

192—A (Chapter 9, Table 9-1) Antilymphocytic globulin (ALG) is a sera directed against T lymphocytes.

Surgery
Must-Know Topics

The following are must-know topics discussed in this review. It would be useful for you to formulate outlines of these subjects since knowledge of the related material will be key to your understanding of the subject and material and for passing the examination.

- Abdominal trauma: treatment

- Appendicitis: signs and symptoms; differential diagnosis

- Blood replacement therapy; transfusion risks

- Burns and injuries from cold: degree and depth; treatment

- Carcinoma of the breast: pathology, diagnosis, routes of metastasis, treatment

- Carcinoma of the colon and rectum: diagnosis, staging, treatment

- Chest trauma: pneumothorax; flail chest; cardiac tamponade; mediastinal masses

(continued)

- Common congenital cardiac lesions: differentiate; prognosis

- Congenital lesions of the head and neck: thyroglossal duct cysts; branchial cleft anomalies

- Coronary artery disease

- Cholecystitis (differentiate acute and chronic), cholelithiasis, and choledocholithiasis: etiology, symptomatology, treatment

- Diverticular disease: symptoms, diagnosis, treatment, management

- Esophageal carcinoma: etiology, diagnosis, treatment

- Fluid and electrolyte imbalances: diagnosis, treatment

- Fractures: specific fractures; dislocations, treatment; compartment syndrome

- Gastroesophageal reflux disease (GERD): management of patient; peptic ulcer disease; indications for surgery

- Hemostasis and coagulation; disseminated intravascular coagulation (DIC)

- Hernia: types, locations, diagnosis, treatment

- Hepatic resection: indications for

- Infections: soft tissue infections

- Inflammatory bowel disease, including ulcerative colitis and Crohn's disease: diagnosis, treatment, management

- Islet cell neoplasms: laboratory tests used to confirm diagnosis

- Malignant tumors of the small intestines

- Pancreatic carcinoma: symptomatology, diagnosis, treatment

- Pancreatitis: etiology, diagnosis, treatment

- Peripheral vascular disease: symptoms, treatment; indications for surgery

- Portal hypertension: portosystemic anastomoses

- Prophylaxis for tetanus; rabies; poisonous snakebites

- Prostate disorders, infections, and cancer: management and treatment

- Pulmonary embolism: method of establishing diagnosis; Virchow's triad

(continued)

- Renal cell carcinoma

- Salivary glands: pleomorphic adenomas; Warthin's tumor

- Shock: types and treatment

- Thyroid cancer: classes, diagnosis, treatment

- Thyroiditis: acute versus chronic; acute suppurative; Hashimoto's, DeQuervain's, Riedel's

- Thyrotoxicosis: diagnosis and treatment of Graves' disease

- Transplantation: graft versus host response; antirejection therapies

- Tumors of the adrenal glands: clinical syndromes of Cushing's syndrome (Cushing's disease), Conn's syndrome

- Tumors of the skin: benign; premalignant and malignant; causes, diagnosis, treatment; management of melanomas

- Wounds: healing process; factors that interfere with healing

Index

Page numbers followed by a *t* refer to tables; those followed by an *f* refer to figures.

Rypins' Intensive Reviews

Series Editor: Edward D. Frohlich, MD

Behavioral Science

Internal Medicine

Surgery

Psychiatry and Behavioral Medicine

FUTURE VOLUMES

Physiology

Pharmacology

Pediatrics

Anatomy

Biochemistry

Microbiology

Pathology

Obstetrics and Gynecology

Community Health